A Guide to
MRCP Part II Ex

A Guide to the
MRCP Part II Examination

R.A. BLACKWOOD
MA, BM BCh, MRCP
Consultant Physician
Wexham Park Hospital, Slough
Honorary Consultant Physician
Hammersmith Hospital
London

T.M.E. DAVIS
BSc, MB BS, DPhil, MRCP
Registrar in Endocrinology
Hammersmith Hospital
London

Blackwell Scientific Publications
OXFORD LONDON EDINBURGH
BOSTON PALO ALTO MELBOURNE

© 1987 by
Blackwell Scientific Publications
Editorial offices:
Osney Mead, Oxford, OX2 0EL
8 John Street, London, WC1N 2ES
23 Ainslie Place, Edinburgh, EH3 6AJ
52 Beacon Street, Boston
  Massachusetts 02108, USA
667 Lytton Avenue, Palo Alto
  California 94301, USA
107 Barry Street, Carlton
  Victoria 3053, Australia

First published 1987

Set by DMB Typesetting (Oxford)
Printed and bound in Great Britain

DISTRIBUTORS

USA
  Year Book Medical Publishers
  35 East Wacker Drive
  Chicago, Illinois 60601

Canada
  The C.V. Mosby Company
  5240 Finch Avenue East,
  Scarborough, Ontario

Australia
  Blackwell Scientific Publications
    (Australia) Pty Ltd
  107 Barry Street
  Carlton, Victoria 3053

British Library
Cataloguing in Publication Data

Blackwood, R.A.
  A guide to the M.R.C.P. Part II
    examination.
  1. Medicine—Problems, exercises,
    etc.
  I. Title   II. Davis, T.M.E.
  610'.76   R834.5

ISBN 0-632-01599-3

Contents

Contents

Preface

Professional examinations such as that for the M.R.C.P. are a test of more than just factual knowledge. Although a candidate's confidence, common sense and consideration for the patient do not come directly from reading, this book gives practical advice on how a thoughtful approach to the patient and his problems might be developed. There is, however, no easy way to exam success and this book should only be used as an adjunct to ward and out-patient clinic experience.

We are grateful to a number of people whose help has been invaluable in the preparation of this book. Valerie Williams spent many hours typing the manuscript and coped admirably with the roughest of drafts. Sanjeev Krishna and other staff on the Medical Unit at Wexham Park Hospital provided valuable criticism of the contents of each chapter, and Derek Griffin produced the high quality clinical photographs. Through the efforts of these people, the task of compiling this book was considerably eased.

R. Blackwood
T. Davis

Introduction:
The Examination in General Outline

Once a candidate has passed the Part I examination for Membership of the Royal College of Physicians (M.R.C.P.), he is then entitled to sit the Part II exam. Part II can only be taken by medical practitioners who have at least eighteen months post-registration experience in approved medical jobs. Testimonials from two sponsors attesting to experience must accompany a candidate's first entry form, with a new testimonial at each successive attempt. A maximum of six attempts are allowed – two at each of the Colleges (Edinburgh, Glasgow and London).

The first section of the Part II exam, the written paper, is the same at each of the three colleges. It consists of a slide, a data interpretation and a case histories section. If a candidate has not failed the written paper irretrievably, he is permitted to proceed to the clinical and oral sections held some weeks later. The clinical exam comprises long and short cases.

The written paper is marked by the examiners of the candidate's college of entry. Examiners for the orals and clinicals are selected to ensure equivalence in standards between the colleges. There is an exchange of examiners to guarantee this, and it is said that the examiners themselves are assessed as to their suitability.

A copy of the examination regulations can be obtained from any of the three colleges, together with future exam dates and fees, and application forms. It is advisable to read the regulations through thoroughly before applying; the colleges will be able to deal with any questions you may have.

The M.R.C.P. is taken during a candidate's general professional training and is designed to select those suitable for higher specialist training in the U.K. In practical terms, it should be a qualification held by practitioners who are competent in managing medical problems in both adults and children with the minimum of supervision.

The following seven chapters are designed to give M.R.C.P. Part II candidates a detailed account of the examination in its current form, as well as hints on preparation for, and approaches to, its various sections.

Chapter 1
The Slide Section

What to expect

The current form of this section is for twenty single or paired slides to be projected in turn for two minutes each; during this time you are required to write down the answers to questions relating to the slide(s). The information requested may be a clinical or pathological diagnosis, a differential diagnosis, the name of a depicted investigation or therapeutic procedure, or a type of radiological abnormality. The question may have a single short answer or several stems. After ninety seconds' projection, a loud warning buzzer rings and a red light comes on at the front of the auditorium, and exactly two minutes later, the next slide comes on to the screen.

As with other sections of the written examination, the regulations are first read out by the chief invigilator and you are asked to check that your answer book is complete. If you have any questions or complaints, it is best to raise them at this stage. A sample slide and set of specimen answers will be projected before the first examination slide.

Candidates will usually be separated by at least one seat from their fellows, and several invigilators are present to discourage cheating. The auditorium lights are set at a bright enough level to allow questions to be read and answers written, yet low enough for detail on the slides to be adequately viewed. Although efforts are made to ensure that everyone has an equivalent view of the screen, there will obviously be differences between the seats, and unfortunately, your examination number dictates where you sit. However, the examiners sit this part of the examination under the same conditions subsequently experienced by the candidates.

At the end of this section, there will be no time to go back and change or complete your answers. When the last slide has been shown, you will have to hand in your answer books promptly.

General preparation

Many slides you are likely to see in the examination will be of material you have already met on the wards or in text books or journals. It is useful to note down details of potential slide subject matter as you meet it, especially if your consultant or registrar comments that it may well appear in the exam. A copy of an X-ray, a duplicate electrocardiogram (E.C.G.) and, if you can obtain them, clinical photographs and slides will all prove useful revision sources.

Your consultants, senior registrars and registrars will probably have their own slide collections, and may be prepared to arrange viewing sessions under examination conditions. Dermatologists, haematologists, ophthalmologists and other specialists in your hospital are worth contacting for the same reason. There are several revision texts on the market with a range of typical exam slides and details of a selection of these books are provided on p. 109.

The slide section will contain a high proportion of straightforward material. It is easy to assume that you are familiar with common conditions and therefore do not need to include them in your revision. However, this assumption can be dangerous. You may think, for example, that the radiologist's report on a chest X-ray of a collapsed right middle lobe states the obvious, but without the report and your history and examination findings, would you be able to interpret the radiological appearances so confidently? The slide section, in common with the clinical part of the exam, could be criticized as artificial as it denies you important background information which would make your answers more assured.

During the examination

When a slide is projected, you may quickly recognize what is being asked. If you are in this fortunate position, double-check the slide and the question before writing down your answer. It is easy to be so relieved at finding one abnormality that other important features on the slide are missed, or there may be a link between abnormalities on a slide which provides the expected answer. For example, a Pagetic clavicle and pleural effusion on a chest X-ray suggest high-output cardiac failure, a diagnosis which would score more marks than one or other abnormality on its own. Once you are satisfied with your answer, there will usually be time for you to read the questions relating to the next slide before it is projected.

If you have no idea as to what you are supposed to be seeing, analyse the projected material systematically. When confronted with a chest X-ray, for example, the time-honoured process of looking specifically at the soft tissues, bones, heart shadow, lung fields and so on will come to your rescue in times of stress. At ninety seconds you should have an idea of what you will put down and, even if you don't, you should write something in the remaining half-minute. It is self-evident that blank answers score nothing, while, if you are fortunate enough to have time to return to difficult questions, you will be able to see how you were thinking at the time the slide was on the screen.

Going back to change your answers can, however make you get out of step with the slides. Panic can set in when you discover that you are two answers behind the number of the slide on the screen. It is therefore very important to check that you are writing each answer down in its correct place. The examiners will make no allowances for candidates who have the right answers out of synchrony with the questions.

Typical examination material

The subject matter which can appear in the slide section is potentially limitless. However, the following headings cover a range of commonly encountered conditions.

Radiographs

It is usual to have at least two or three X-rays in the exam. The chest X-ray appears most often and some of the more subtle abnormalities include (see Figure 1.1):
- apical pneumothorax
- azygous lobe
- cervical rib
- dextrocardia
- gas under the diaphragm
- hiatus hernia
- hilar lymphadenopathy
- old fractures/thoracotomies

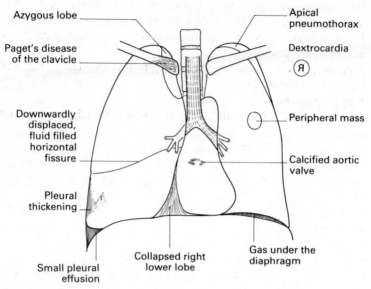

Azygous lobe

Paget's disease of the clavicle

Downwardly displaced, fluid filled horizontal fissure

Pleural thickening

Small pleural effusion

Collapsed right lower lobe

Apical pneumothorax

Dextrocardia

Peripheral mass

Calcified aortic valve

Gas under the diaphragm

Figure 1.1. Schematic diagram of a selection of commonly encountered chest X-ray abnormalities.

- Paget's disease of clavicle/humerus
- peripheral lung/pleural lesions
- rib notching
- silicone breast implants
- unilateral mastectomy
- widened mediastinum

In some of these cases, a lateral chest X-ray would be of great help but is seldom shown.

Abdominal and pelvic X-rays do not appear as often, but it is worth looking for the following if there is nothing obvious at first:
- abnormal renal size/outline
- calcification (aorta, kidney, pancreas, bladder, fibroid)
- dermoid cyst (e.g. a tooth)
- heavy metal injection sites
- Looser's zones
- loss of psoas shadows
- Paget's disease of pelvis/femora
- radio-opaque stones (urinary tract, gallbladder)
- sacroiliitis

Other plain X-rays which may appear include films of the skull, hands and feet, long bones and vertebral column. You should be

familiar with the more common abnormalities seen on these X-rays and on the following specialized radiological investigations:
• angiography (carotid, coeliac, coronary, renal and pulmonary arteriograms, and venography)
• barium studies (swallow and meal, follow-through, small and large bowel enemata)
• bronchography
• computerised axial tomography (CT scan: cranial, thoracic and abdominal)
• echocardiography (two-dimensional, M-mode)
• gallbladder and biliary tract investigations (oral cholecystogram, intravenous cholangiogram, endoscopic retrograde cholangio-pancreaticogram)
• isotope scanning (bone, brain, liver, thyroid, ventilation/perfusion)
• lymphangiography
• myelography/radiculography
• renal tract investigations (intravenous urography, antegrade and retrograde pyelography)
• ultrasonography (upper abdominal and pelvic)
Newer techniques such as digital subtraction angiography, magnetic resonance imaging and radiolabelled white cell scans may also be included.

Dermatological slides

These occur regularly. If a skin condition is not immediately recognizable, a 'surgical sieve' may help you:
• *Infective* – bacterial (erysipelas, impetigo, meningococcaemia, syphilis), viral (herpes zoster, orf, measles), fungal (tinea versicolor, candida) and parasitic (scabies, larva migrans, vagabond's disease).
• *Vascular* – ischaemic and venous ulcers, vasculitis (including splinter haemorrhages and nail fold infarcts) and purpura.
• *Neoplastic* – ranging from primary tumours (squamous and basal cell carcinomata, melanoma, keratoacanthoma, subungual fibroma) to acanthosis nigricans, dermatomyositis and neurofibromatosis.
• *Degenerative* – including solar keratosis and senile warts.
• *Metabolic and hormonal* – including insulin lipodystrophy, xanthelasmata/xanthomata, glucagonoma rash, pre-tibial myxoedema and necrobiosis lipoidica diabeticorum.

- *Traumatic* – including keloid scars, dermatitis artefacta and intravenous drug abuse.
- *Autoimmune* – including systemic lupus erythematosus, discoid lupus, systemic sclerosis.
- *Iatrogenic* – such as drug eruptions and steroid-induced skin changes.
- *Idiopathic* – including conditions associated with specific diseases (lichen planus, vitiligo, lupus pernio, pyoderma gangrenosum, erythema nodosum, psoriasis).

This is by no means a comprehensive list but provides a means of finding the most likely diagnosis.

Haematology

It pays to be familiar with common blood film and/or bone marrow appearances of the following:
- acanthocytosis
- acute and chronic leukaemias
- aplastic anaemia
- atypical lymphocytes
- carcinomatous marrow infiltration
- common red cell morphological abnormalities
- lead poisoning
- leucoerythroblastic blood picture
- malaria, leishmaniasis, trypanosomiasis
- megaloblastic anaemia
- multiple myeloma
- post-splenectomy
- sideroblastic anaemia

Ophthalmology

Covers slides of the eyelids, sclerae, cornea, iris, pupil and fundus. Examples of commonly encountered abnormalities include:
- Argyll Robertson pupils
- band keratopathy
- blue sclerae
- cataracts of all types
- cherry-red macula
- cholesterol embolus
- choroidoretinitis

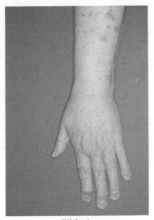

Slide 1

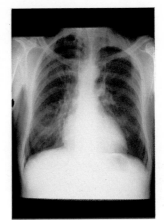

Slide 2

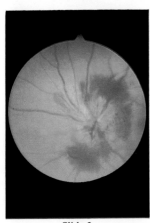

Slide 3

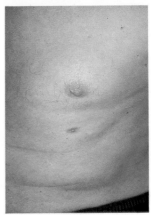

Slide 4

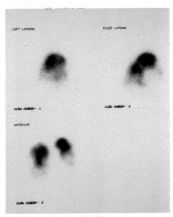

Slide 5

Plate 1

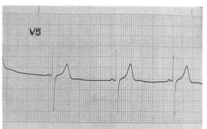

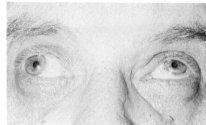

Slide 6

Slide 7

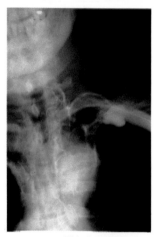

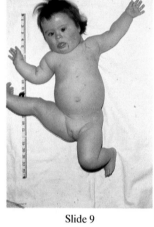

Slide 8

Slide 9

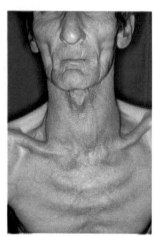

Slide 10

Plate 2

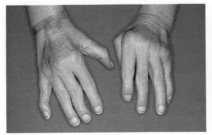

Slide 11

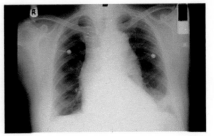

Slide 12

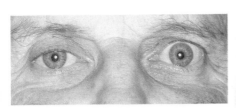

Slide 13

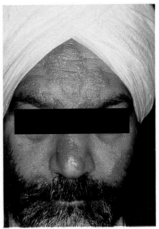

Slide 14

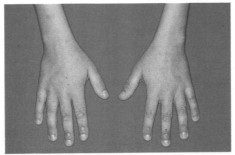

Slide 15

Plate 3

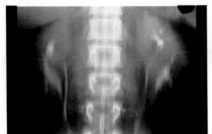

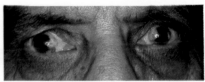

Slide 17

Slide 16

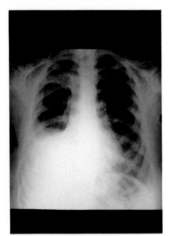

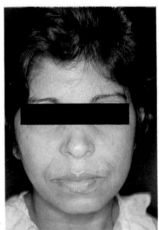

Slide 18

Slide 19

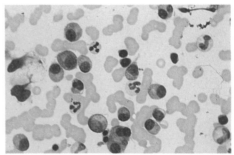

Slide 20

Plate 4

- diabetic retinopathy
- glaucoma
- Holmes-Adie pupils
- hypertensive retinopathy
- iritis and hypopyon
- Kayser-Fleischer rings
- lipaemia retinalis
- optic atrophy
- papilloedema
- retinal artery and vein occlusions
- retinitis pigmentosa
- Roth spots
- scleritis and episcleritis
- sicca syndrome

You must be able to distinguish between retinal abnormalities which appear similar (e.g. hypertensive retinopathy and central retinal vein occlusion).

Syndromes

May be discernible from a view of the whole patient (e.g. Turner's and Kleinfelter's) or from a part of the body (e.g. the hyperelastic skin of Ehlers-Danlos and the hands of Down's). These are usually straightforward.

Hands and feet

There is considerable overlap with dermatology; with psoriatic rash and arthropathy, splinter haemorrhages, scabies and vitiligo being examples of commonly-encountered conditions. The hands of rheumatoid arthritis, acromegaly and arachnodactyly are also exam favourites. The nails may be the focus of attention in which case bear in mind:
- brown crescents of renal failure
- clubbing
- leuconychia
- onycholysis
- paronychia
- psoriasis
- yellow nail syndrome

Neurological abnormalities are often shown in slides of the hands including:

- carpal tunnel syndrome
- carpo-pedal spasm
- T1 motorneuron lesions
- ulnar and radial nerve lesions

Remember that the feet can display the same pathology as the hands (rheumatoid foot with nodules for example) and may be shown in an effort to make the diagnosis less obvious.

Pathology

You will either be shown a gross specimen (such as an atrial myxoma or a hypernephroma) or a histological abnormality (such as subtotal villous atrophy or a caseating granuloma). It is worth going through a pathology text to reacquaint yourself with common conditions which are also clinically important.

Electrocardiograms

Are more usually encountered in the data interpretation section of the exam where they are bound to have multiple abnormalities. In the slide section, single diagnoses are usual, including:

- dextrocardia
- hypothermia
- myocarditis/pericarditis
- Wolff-Parkinson-White syndrome

Others

Urine specimens, endoscopic appearances and dystonic posturing are examples of potential slide section subject matter which do not fall clearly into the above broad subject headings. Again, it is imperative that you have had a wide exposure across the specialities, even if this has in part been through text books and journals.

Trial examination questions

(see plates 1–4 for colour slides)

Slide 1:   What is the diagnosis?

Slide 2:   What abnormal radiological features are present?
What is the diagnosis?

Slide 3:   What is the diagnosis?

Slide 4:   What feature is present?
What treatment would you recommend?

Slide 5:   What investigation is shown?
What is the probable diagnosis?

Slide 6:   What is the diagnosis?

Slide 7:   This patient has been asked to look straight upwards.
What is the diagnosis?

Slide 8:   What radiological investigation is shown?
What abnormalities are present?

Slide 9:   What is the diagnosis?

Slide 10:   This patient presented in high-output cardiac failure.
What is the diagnosis?

Slide 11:   What are the diagnoses?

Slide 12:   What abnormalities are present?
What is the diagnosis?

Slide 13:   What abnormality is present?
What is the most likely cause?

Slide 14:   What is the diagnosis?
What treatment would you consider?

Slide 15:   What feature is present?

Slide 16:   What investigation is shown?
What abnormality is present?

Slide 17:   This patient has emigrated from India. What is the
diagnosis?

Slide 18:   What abnormalities are present?

Slide 19: What abnormal feature is present?
          Which investigation would best confirm the diagnosis?

Slide 20: What is the diagnosis?
          List three investigations, the results of which might con-
          firm the diagnosis.

Answers

Slide 1: The presence of psoriasis and an arthropathy involving the distal interphalangeal joints confirm the diagnosis of *psoriatic arthropathy*.

Slide 2: There is an opacity at the left apex and the left second rib is eroded. There is also a fracture of the ninth rib on the right. These features suggest the presence of a *Pancoast tumour with metastases*.

Slide 3: This fundal photograph shows *the retinopathy of malignant hypertension* as evidenced by subhyaloid and flame-shaped haemorrhages, and by papilloedema.

Slide 4: This slide shows an *accessory nipple*. No treatment is necessary.

Slide 5: This lung perfusion scan shows multiple areas of decreased uptake, consistent with *pulmonary emboli*.

Slide 6: There is a very short P–R interval without any deformation of the QRS complex. These features are consistent with a diagnosis of *Lown-Ganong-Levine syndrome*.

Slide 7: This patient's right eye is deviated to the right and is not as elevated as the left. There is no ptosis on the right. A *partial right occulomotor nerve palsy with pupillary sparing* would explain these features.

Slide 8: This venogram shows obstruction to flow through the left axillary and subclavian veins with collaterals present. This is *thrombosis of the left subclavian vein*.

Slide 9: This baby has all the features of *Down's syndrome* (hypotonicity, macroglossia, epicanthic folds, single palmar crease).

Slide 10: The presence of a goitre and high-output cardiac failure makes *Graves' disease* the likely diagnosis.

Slide 11: These are the hands of *rheumatoid arthritis* (swan-necking, swollen metacarpophalangeal joints, ulnar deviation and wasting of the small muscles of the hands). The brown crescents visible on each of the nails suggest either *chronic renal failure* or *congestive cardiac failure*.

Slide 12: The widened mediastinum, deviated trachea and left basal shadowing point to a diagnosis of *dissecting aortic aneurysm*.

Slide 13: The patient has a *right-sided ptosis* which, in the absence of other signs, is usually congenital in origin.

Slide 14: This patient has *lupus pernio* which can be treated with chloroquine or corticosteroids.

Slide 15: *Garrod's pads* are present over the knuckles on both hands.

Slide 16: This tomogram of an intravenous urogram shows *bilaterally duplex collecting systems*.

Slide 17: This man has *bilateral pterygia*.

Slide 18: There is *right mid and upper zone fibrosis* together with *right lower zone consolidation*.

Slide 19: This is the butterfly rash of *systemic lupus erythematosus*, best confirmed by a high antibody titre to double-stranded DNA.

Slide 20: This bone marrow aspirate shows a preponderance of plasma cells, confirming a diagnosis of *multiple myeloma*. Serum electrophoresis, urinalysis for Bence-Jones proteins and a skeletal survey are other important investigations which aid in diagnosis.

Chapter 2
Case Histories

What to expect

In the case histories (or 'grey cases') section of the examination, there are four to six questions to be answered within 55 minutes. The questions to be answered usually have several stems and relate to a description of a clinical case complete with the results of investigations. The first part of each question usually asks for a diagnosis or differential diagnosis of the case. You may then be asked what further investigations are indicated and what lines of management you would pursue.

Because the cases are 'grey', there are no single correct answers. However, there will be some answers that are much more appropriate than others and marks are allocated on this basis – only the answer which is considered the best by the examiners will receive full marks.

Before the examination starts, the regulations are read out and you are asked to check that your answer book is complete. The questions appear on the left-hand pages and there are one or two lines for the answers on the page opposite. No rough paper is provided but candidates may make notes on the question page. Normal ranges for common variables (such as plasma urea and electrolyte concentrations) are not usually given. However, the results of more unusual investigations are accompanied by reference ranges for comparison.

The complexity of the grey cases varies considerably. There may be almost a page of history and examination findings for some questions and a brief paragraph for others. The lists of investigations (not all of which are necessarily relevant) can be long or even absent. Some questions require a single answer while others consist of several questions relating to phases of a patient's complex clinical course. As a result, it is difficult to know how much time to allocate to each question though the 55 minutes allowed is sufficient for most candidates to finish the paper without undue haste.

15

General preparation

Clinical acumen depends on background knowledge and experience, and the case histories section is arguably the part of the M.R.C.P. exam which is the best test of this. You will doubtless have looked after patients whose condition required a reasoned and logical approach to obtain a diagnosis and these types of cases are ideal preparation. It is possible, in retrospect, to check whether your investigations and management were justified and appropriate. Such cases are often presented at hospital or departmental meetings and it is well worth attending these.

It is wise to keep up with the main journals. Reports of new clinical syndromes or unusual presentations of familiar diseases (Legionnaires' disease and toxic shock syndrome for example) can form the basis of a grey case. It should also be remembered that paediatric, obstetric and surgical cases with medical problems appear in the exam. There are revision texts which have a wide range of cases in examination format and these are a useful revision source. Nevertheless it is self-evident that the wards and outpatient clinics are the best places to develop the diagnostic skills and competence in patient management that this section of the exam is designed to assess.

During the examination

It pays to read through the clinical information and investigations with great care, underlining main points and annotating where necessary. In some questions, there may be one or two pieces of information which are the key to the correct answers and it is important not to skip over them. If the reference ranges are provided, it is good practice to take heed of them. You may think you know whether a particular result is normal or abnormal, but unfamiliar units of measurement and laboratory techniques may have been used to obtain it. The questions themselves are unambiguous but, as in any exam, you should be careful to answer what is asked.

The space for answers is more than adequate for the correct response – if you find you are writing down more than the examiners expect, your answer may be over-elaborate or even wrong. When you are satisfied with your answer, it is sensible to check that it is in the right place, especially if you have crossed out several previous attempts. Indeed, if you are unsure about an answer, it is probably better to jot down the possibilities on the question page, and to come back and decide on the best alternative when you have completed another question, or at the end of the exam.

Your answers should be as specific as possible: for example, 'Crohn's disease of the terminal ileum' is more accurate than just 'Crohn's disease', or 'right posterior cerebral artery embolus' much more informative than 'cerebrovascular accident'. Words without specific meaning such as 'lesion' are best avoided, as are *all* abbreviations no matter how commonly used. Units of measurement should not be omitted if a quantitative answer is required. Again, blank answers score no marks and it is always preferable to write something down no matter how feeble an attempt it might seem.

Typical examination material

The scope of the grey cases is broad. However, the range of examination material encountered in the data interpretation section (see Chapter 3) also covers the majority of grey cases you will meet. The following are examples of typical questions together with model answers.

Trial examination questions

Case history 1

A 31-year-old woman is brought into Casualty one evening by ambulance. She is unconscious and unaccompanied. On examination she is afebrile but tachypnoeic; she has a regular pulse rate of 120 beats/minute but otherwise the cardiovascular system is normal. There are fine crackles at both lung bases on auscultation of the chest. Abdominal examination reveals no abnormality. She responds to painful stimuli and her plantar responses are extensor; there are no focal neurological signs. At the end of the examination, she has a grand mal convulsion which responds rapidly to intravenous diazepam.

Haemoglobin concentration	13.9 g/dl
White cell count	11.0×10^9/l
Mean corpuscular volume	82 fl
Erythrocyte sedimentation rate	18 mm/hour
Serum concentrations:	
bilirubin	10 μmol/l
aspartate aminotransferase	20 iU/l
total protein	70 g/l
albumin	35 g/l
calcium	2.30 mmol/l
Plasma concentrations:	
sodium	141 mmol/l
potassium	3.0 mmol/l
bicarbonate	10 mmol/l

Question: What is the most likely diagnosis?
Question: What three other diagnoses are also possible?
Question: What four other investigations would you request urgently?
Question: What therapeutic manoeuvre may be necessary?

    With treatment, her clinical condition improves overnight but the next morning she has a persistent sinus tachycardia and complains of blurred vision.
Question: What other diagnosis would explain these abnormalities?

Answer

This lady has a *metabolic acidosis*. She also has hypokalaemia and presumptive evidence of pulmonary oedema. These features make *salicylate poisoning* the most likely diagnosis, but *diabetic ketoacidosis*, *acute renal failure* and *lactic acidosis* must also be considered. Other causes of a metabolic acidosis (such as renal tubular acidosis and diarrhoea) are less likely.

It is essential to know the results of a *drug screen* on blood and urine including a plasma salicylate level, *arterial blood gas analysis*, *urea and creatinine concentrations* and a *plasma glucose concentration*. Urinalysis for glucose and ketones, microscopy and culture of the urine and a blood lactate level are useful but not necessary to make the diagnosis and initiate treatment in this case.

She may require *alkaline diuresis* if her salicylate level is high – haemodialysis is usually reserved for very high levels and is carried out in specialist centres.

Her subsequent clinical course suggests that she may have taken a *tricyclic antidepressant overdose* in addition to the salicylate, as she has evidence of cardiotoxicity and anticholinergic side-effects.

Case history 2

A 38-year-old woman from Antigua presents to outpatients with a four month history of malaise, weight loss and arthralgia. She also complains of intermittent dyspnoea, dry cough and sore eyes. A year previously, she had apparently presented to a hospital in Antigua with similar symptoms and was treated with a six month course of at least two medications. One of these was the same drug as a neighbour was taking for tuberculosis. She could not remember the names of these drugs but her symptoms improved while she was on treatment. She smokes 20 cigarettes per day and drinks the occasional measure of spirits. On examination she is pallid and pyrexial with both a smooth liver edge and tip of spleen palpable on deep inspiration.

Haemoglobin concentration	10.9 g/dl
Mean corpuscular volume	63 fl
Mean corpuscular haemoglobin concentration	32 g/dl
White cell count	$9.8 \times 10^9/l$
Platelet count	$175 \times 10^9/l$
Erythrocyte sedimentation rate	49 mm/hour

Plasma concentrations:

sodium	139 mmol/l
potassium	3.8 mmol/l
urea	8.9 mmol/l
bicarbonate	27 mmol/l

Serum concentrations:

bilirubin	20 μmol/l
aspartate aminotransferase	45 iU/l
total protein	76 g/l
albumin	29 g/l
calcium	2.69 mmol/l

Question: What two distinct diagnoses would you consider?
Question: What single investigation would you request in order to best confirm the diagnosis in each case?
Question: What treatment would you consider?

Answer

The combination of systemic and respiratory symptoms, together with dry eyes, mild splenomegaly and hypercalcaemia suggest the diagnosis of *sarcoidosis* though a *lymphoma* may also explain these features. Sarcoidosis does not respond to antituberculous treatment but this may be given in addition to corticosteroids where there is a high risk of exposure to tuberculosis in patients who either have extensive pulmonary disease or who are tuberculin-positive. However, *tuberculosis* on its own seems an unlikely diagnosis in this case.

The microcytic anaemia with a normal mean corpuscular haemoglobin concentration is suggestive of a haemoglobinopathy such as *sickle-cell trait*. Indeed, sarcoidosis has a much increased incidence in black people in whom sickle-cell disease must always be considered as an explanation for anaemia. It could well be that this woman is black as she is from the West Indies.

A *Kveim-Siltzbach skin test* and *haemoglobin electrophoresis* will best confirm the diagnosis in each case.

This woman has systemic symptoms and ocular involvement, and consideration should be given for treating her with *oral corticosteroids*.

Case history 3

A 69-year-old man who had recently lost his wife attended his general practitioner on the insistence of his daughter. He lived alone and was finding it difficult to cope. He complained that he had developed arthritis in his joints and that he was troubled by pain in his neck together with intermittent headache. He admitted to weight loss of about one stone over the previous month. He also thought that he needed new glasses as his vision had been recently deteriorating. He was taking amitriptyline 25 mg nocte but no other medication when seen.

Question: What three diagnoses are possible on the above history?

On examination, his pulse rate was regular at 70 beats/minute and his supine blood pressure was 170/95 mmHg. His heart sounds were normal and there was no evidence of cardiac failure. There were no abnormal findings in the respiratory system and his abdomen was soft with no organ enlargement or masses palpable. A quick neurological examination of his limbs revealed no abnormalities.

Question: What three other aspects of the physical examination would be important in allowing the correct diagnosis to be made?

Question: What single investigation would you first request?

Answer

This man's symptoms could be a manifestation of *depression*. However, *giant cell arteritis* should always be considered in a patient with failing vision and arthralgia/myalgia, while he might also have *occult malignancy* or widespread *osteoarthritis*. *Osteomalacia* is also a diagnostic possibility.

Palpation of the temporal arteries, *fundoscopy* and *examination of the joints* are important aspects of physical examination in this case.

The *erythrocyte sedimentation rate* (ESR) should be determined urgently and, if it is markedly raised, high dose corticosteroids should be given.

Case history 4

A 52-year-old Caucasian male was admitted to the intensive care unit. Six weeks prior to admission he had been involved in a road traffic accident in Zaire and had undergone emergency laparotomy. A ruptured left hemidiaphragm, ruptured spleen, large retroperitoneal haematoma and an infarcted colon at the splenic flexure were found. His diaphragm was repaired and his spleen removed; the infarcted bowel was resected and a colostomy was fashioned. He required a ten-unit blood transfusion. He was successfully treated for a wound infection in the immediate postoperative period but had again become pyrexial two days prior to his flight back to the U.K. He was taken to hospital straight from Heathrow airport.

On examination he had a temperature of 40.2°C. His blood pressure was 80/60 mmHg and his pulse was 130/minute and weak. There was fresh blood in the colostomy bag and a large haematoma in his left antecubital fossa at the site of a recent venepuncture. There was dullness to percussion and absent breath sounds at the left lung base, but otherwise examination of the cardiovascular and respiratory systems was unremarkable. His abdomen was generally tender to palpation.

Question: What is the most likely condition underlying his recent deterioration?
Question: What complication may well be present?

The laboratory staff refuse to process any blood samples from this patient.

Question: Suggest a reason for this.
Question: What three investigations not involving blood would be of help in confirming the primary diagnosis?

Answer

This unfortunate man has developed a marked pyrexia following recent abdominal surgery involving the bowel. He has abdominal tenderness and signs of a left-sided pleural effusion both of which are consistent with a *subphrenic abscess*. His bleeding tendency could be a manifestation of *disseminated intravascular coagulation* complicating the abscess. A *left basal pneumonia* might also be an explanation for his clinical condition. Because he has come from Central Africa, *a viral haemorrhagic fever* must be considered and *malaria* excluded. Indeed, the laboratory staff may have refused to handle his samples because of the risk of the presence of a *Category A pathogen* in his blood, especially as he has had a transfusion as an emergency. The risk of *Acquired Immunodeficiency Syndrome* (AIDS) may also deter the laboratory staff from handling his blood but there are now well-established procedures in use for samples from patients with AIDS.

An *ultrasound scan, gallium scan, radiolabelled white cell scan* and *abdominal CT scan* are investigations which would be helpful in demonstrating a sub-diaphragmatic collection.

Case history 5

An unmarried 54-year-old school teacher was admitted with weakness in his right arm and leg. With some difficulty he was able to give a history. Three years previously he was found to have a lymphoma and received both chemotherapy and radiotherapy; he did not bother to attend follow-up after the first year. For the four weeks prior to admission, he had noticed increasing weakness of his right limbs together with difficulty in making his students understand him during lessons. He also complained of a constant headache. He was a non-smoker and teetotaller and on no medication when admitted.

Physical examination revealed no cardiovascular or respiratory abnormalities, and his abdomen was soft with no organ enlargement or palpable masses. There was moderate right-sided weakness and hyper-reflexia, and the right plantar response was extensor. Fundoscopy revealed no papilloedema but a raised, pigmented area of approximately one disc diameter as found above the right macula. Visual fields were full to confrontation and the cranial nerves were otherwise normal.

Haemoglobin concentration	11.0 g/dl
Mean corpuscular volume	81 fl
Mean corpuscular haemoglobin concentration	33 g/dl
White cell count (normal differential)	6.7×10^9/l
Erythrocyte sedimentation rate	82 mm/hour
Plasma concentrations:	
sodium	131 mmol/l
potassium	3.7 mmol/l
bicarbonate	22 mmol/l
urea	10.8 mmol/l
creatinine	130 μmol/l ·
Serum concentrations:	
bilirubin	30 μmol/l
aspartate aminotransferase	88 iU/l
alkaline phosphatase	457 iU/l
total protein	64 g/l
albumin	26 g/l

IgG	8.0 g/l
IgA	4.2 g/l
IgM	1.0 g/l

Chest X-ray: normal

Electrocardiogram: partial right bundle branch block.

Urinalysis: ketones +

Question: Give the three most likely causes for this recent deterioration.

Question: Give three other investigations which would facilitate making the correct diagnosis.

Answer

This man has evidence of pathology in his left cerebral hemisphere with upper motor neuron signs in his right limbs and a probable expressive dysphasia. Although he has had a lymphoma in the past, the picture is one of a space-occupying lesion, something which is unusual for *lymphomatous CNS involvement*. He has abnormal liver function tests, is mildly anaemic and has a raised ESR. There is also a pigmented area on his right retina, making a *cerebral metastasis from a melanoma* a distinct possibility. The other malignancy which commonly metastasises to the brain in males is a *bronchial carcinoma* but there is little evidence for this diagnosis here. Other diagnoses that could be considered are *cerebral abscess*, *progressive multifocal leucoencephalopathy* and *cerebrovascular disease* but all are less likely than disseminated melanoma.

A *cranial CT scan*, if necessary with enhancement, should be performed, as well as a *liver ultrasound scan* proceeding to a *liver biopsy* for tissue diagnosis.

Chapter 3
Data Interpretation

What to expect

This section of the examination consists of ten questions to be answered within 45 minutes. The questions usually have several parts and relate to a short clinical description followed by the results of selected investigations. The data presented are diverse, from E.C.G.s and lung function tests to acid-base studies and haematological profiles.

The data interpretation paper follows on immediately after the grey cases. Candidates who finish the case histories before the 55 minutes allowed may go on and start the data interpretation section early. However, there is usually plenty of time available to answer all ten questions in the 45 minutes. The questions contain a comparable amount of clinical and laboratory information, and there is usually a single correct answer.

The layout of the question/answer book is the same as that for the case histories. No reference ranges accompany commonly encountered variables and the space provided for answers is limited to one or two lines. Quantitative answers may be required but the necessary calculations will usually be simple.

General preparation

Most candidates will have had plenty of experience analysing the results of 'routine' investigations such as full blood counts and E.C.G.s. However, it is good exam practice to interpret such data in cases where you are 'blind' to the background clinical information. You may be surprised at your errors and omissions.

More 'specialized' investigations such as pituitary stimulation tests and cardiac catheterization may be unfamiliar to you if you have not had clinical experience in the relevant field. Revision texts are a useful source of examples of these tests which can also appear in journal case reports. Large text books are obviously the place to find the theory behind and technical details of these investigations. Indeed, a proper understanding of the pathophysiology assessed by a particular test will be invaluable in interpreting the results.

29

During the examination

Your approach to the data interpretation section should be the same as that for the case histories – to put down carefully reasoned answers which are neither over-elaborate nor laced with vague terms and abbreviations. Candidates find that they 'fret' over the answers much less than they did during the case histories section because there are no 'shades of grey'. Again, *all* questions should be attempted, even those that you think you have little chance of getting right.

Typical examination material

A broad cross-section of the type of material which appears in this section of the examination is detailed below by system.

Cardiology

Electrocardiograms. As mentioned in Chapter 1, these will almost certainly have multiple abnormalities. If you are asked for less features than you can identify, put the most clinically important ones down first (complete heart block ahead of borderline voltage criteria for left ventricular hypertrophy for example). You should be conversant with:
• conduction abnormalities (first, second and third degree heart block; bundle branch block)
• infarction patterns (including ventricular aneurysms)
• arrhythmias (tachyarrhythmias and bradyarrhythmias)
• pulmonary embolism
• left and right ventricular hypertrophy
• interpretation of the post-exercise E.C.G.
Questions relating to the E.C.G.s displayed usually require a diagnosis (Wolff-Parkinson-White syndrome for example) and/or treatment (such as an inferior myocardial infarction with complete heart block requiring temporary pacing).

Data from cardiac catheterization. It is wise to learn the normal ranges for pressures and oxygen saturation within each of the cardiac chambers and large vessels (see Figure 3.1). This will facilitate interpretation of catheter data from patients with:
• atrial and ventricular septal defects

- valvular disease (stenosis and/or incompetence)
- systemic and pulmonary hypertension
- constrictive pericarditis

Complex syndromes (e.g. Fallot's tetralogy and other congenital heart lesions), which are usually a combination of such abnormalities, can also appear.

General. Data interpretation questions can be framed around other cardiological conditions including:
- infective endocarditis
- rheumatic fever
- cardiomyopathies
- post myocardial infarction (Dressler's) syndrome

Neurology

CSF findings. You should be familiar with the normal ranges for concentrations of glucose and protein in cerebrospinal fluid as well as normal cell counts. CSF data consistent with the following diagnoses may appear in the exam:
- meningitis: bacterial (including tuberculosis and syphilis), viral, fungal, carcinomatous.

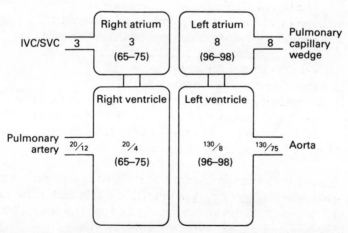

Figure 3.1. Schematic diagram showing normal intracardiac pressures in mm Hg and, in brackets, percentage oxygen saturations.

- subarachnoid haemorrhage
- Guillain-Barré syndrome
- multiple sclerosis (MS)
- Froin's syndrome

Electrophysiological tests. These very seldom appear in the examination but neurological questions may contain basic data from the following specialized investigations:
- electroencephalography (EEG)
- evoked responses (visual, auditory and somatosensory)
- electromyography (EMG)

General. Many diseases may present with neurological symptoms and signs, whilst focal signs will allow localization of a neurological lesion. Both these situations may be incorporated into data interpretation questions.

Respiratory medicine

Lung function tests. The complexity of lung function test data varies with the type of investigation used. These include:
- simple spirometry (peak flow and Vitalograph measurements)
- detailed assessment of lung volumes (including total lung capacity, vital capacity, functional residual capacity and tidal volume: see Figure 3.2)

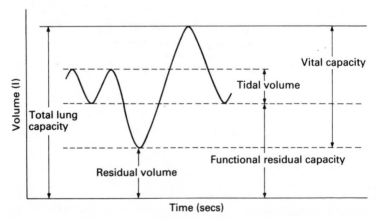

Figure 3.2. Spirometric tracing showing lung volumes and their relationships.

The two basic types of defect detected by spirometry are (see Figure 3.3):

• restrictive (including fibrosing aveolitis, pulmonary infiltrations, pleural effusion and thickening, pneumoconioses)

• obstructive (chronic bronchitis and emphysema, asthma)

Other data which may be included are:

• gas diffusion studies (transfer factor) which can be affected by respiratory and cardiac disease, and variations in the haematocrit

• flow-volume loops (see Figure 3.4)

General. Other respiratory investigations which may be used in data interpretation questions are:

• analysis of pleural fluid (cell count, protein concentration and glucose concentration in conditions such as rheumatoid arthritis, heart failure, pulmonary embolism and pneumonia)

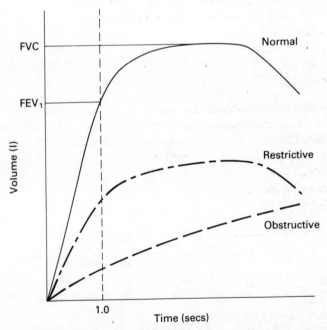

Figure 3.3. Vitalograph tracings showing restrictive and obstructive defects. The forced vital capacity (FVC) and forced expiratory volume in the first second (FEV_1) for the normal tracing are shown. For a restrictive defect, FEV_1/FVC is >70%; for an obstructive defect this ratio is <70%.

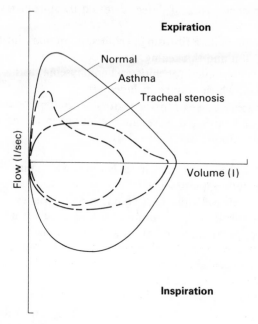

Figure 3.4. Flow-volume curves in a normal individual, and in patients with tracheal stenosis and asthma.

- sweat test (cystic fibrosis)
- analysis of bronchial lavage cell counts (sarcoidosis and fibrosing alveolitis)

Renal medicine

Plasma and urine biochemistry. Data interpretation questions on renal diseases usually require analysis of the following investigations alone or in combination:
- plasma urea, electrolytes, creatinine and osmolality
- urinary urea, electrolytes, creatinine and osmolality
- creatinine clearance and other estimates of glomerular filtration rate (GFR)
- plasma and urinary urate concentrations
- urinary protein excretion (with selectivity)
- urinary calcium excretion
- plasma renin and aldosterone concentrations

• presence of unusual substances in the urine (including amino-aciduria, Bence-Jones proteins and haemosiderin)

It is important to identify the following conditions from bio-chemical data and relevant clinical information:

• acute, chronic and acute-on-chronic renal failure and their many causes
• nephrotic syndrome (when the plasma cholesterol concentration may also be supplied)
• diabetes insipidus
• renal tubular acidosis (conventionally types 1 and 2)
• salt-losing nephritis
• Fanconi's syndrome (congenital and adult forms)
• renal glycosuria
• ureterosigmoidostomy

Urine microscopy. Microscopy of the urine for cells, casts, crystals and organisms may be valuable in the diagnosis of the above conditions but also in:

• renal tract infections (including tuberculosis)
• renal stones
• analgesic nephropathy
• polycystic kidneys
• renal tract tumours
• benign prostatic hypertrophy

Acid-base status. Will be covered fully under 'Metabolic medicine'.

General. Renal investigations may be used to aid diagnosis of a range of multisystem disorders such as infective endocarditis and sickle-cell disease (haematuria), myeloma (Bence-Jones proteinuria and renal failure) and Legionnaires' disease (hyponatraemia, haematuria and mild proteinuria).

Gastroenterology

Liver function tests. The results of these are commonly quoted in data interpretation questions of diverse types, but some of the gastroenterological conditions in which liver function tests are important when arriving at the correct diagnosis include:

• primary biliary cirrhosis (PBC: an antimitochondrial antibody titre may also be supplied)

• acute and chronic hepatitis (when an anti-smooth muscle antibody titre may aid diagnosis of chronic active hepatitis)
• congenital hyperbilirubinaemias (Gilbert's, Crigler-Najjar, Dubin-Johnson and Rotor syndromes)
• Wilson's disease (with serum copper and ceruloplasmin concentrations)
• drug-induced cholestasis

Tests of malabsorption. It pays to be familiar with the following investigations:
• xylose absorption test
• three-day faecal fat excretion
• C^{14}glycocholic breath test
• Schilling test
• pancreatic function tests (the secretin/pancreozymin test and Lundh test meal)

General. Other tests which may appear in this section of the written exam include:
• pentagastrin test
• insulin hypoglycaemia test
• fasting plasma gastrin concentration
• bromsulphthalein (BSP) retention test
• hepatitis antigen status

Metabolic medicine and endocrinology

Acid-base balance. It is wise to be familiar with the normal ranges (in SI units) of arterial pH, Pao_2 $Paco_2$, as well as the meaning of the terms 'standard bicarbonate', 'base excess' or 'deficit' and 'anion gap'. The four basic abnormalities you will be expected to identify are (see Figure 3.5):
• respiratory acidosis and alkalosis
• metabolic acidosis and alkalosis
Combinations of the above can appear in the exam (e.g. a mixed respiratory and metabolic acidosis in a patient with severe pneumonia complicated by diabetic ketoacidosis), when compensatory mechanisms may be in operation.
The two types of lactic acidosis which may form the basis of a data interpretation question are:
• Type A (with shock or severe hypoxia)
• Type B (in the absence of shock)

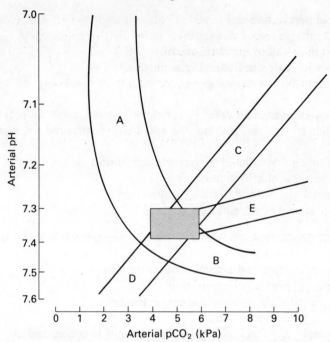

Figure 3.5. Acid-base status showing (A) metabolic acidosis, (B) metabolic alkalosis, (C) respiratory acidosis, (D) respiratory alkalosis, (E) compensated respiratory acidosis.

Water and electrolyte metabolism. The recognition of water excess and deficiency or sodium excess and deficiency is facilitated by a knowledge of the normal ranges for plasma osmolarity (and its quick calculation from the plasma sodium, potassium, urea and glucose concentrations):

$$2 [Na^+ + K^+] + [Urea] + [Glucose]$$

and urinary osmolarity. You should know the causes of
• hypo- and hypernatraemia
• hypo- and hyperkalaemia
• hypo- and hypercalcaemia
• hypo- and hypercalciuria
• syndrome of inappropriate anti-diuretic hormone excretion (SIADH)
The investigation of polyuria and polydipsia which is not due to diabetes mellitus or renal impairment usually entails interpretation of

- fluid deprivation test
- vasopressin test

which may lead to the diagnosis of

- diabetes insipidus (cranial or nephrogenic)
- compulsive overdrinking

Hyperlipidaemias. The Friedrickson classification should be familiar to you and you may be asked to interpret the following data:

- serum cholesterol and triglyceride concentrations
- lipoprotein electrophoresis
- plasma glucose and urate concentrations
- appearance of stored serum

Metabolic bone disease. You may be presented with data such as:

- serum calcium and albumin concentrations
- serum phosphate concentration
- serum alkaline phosphatase concentration
- urinary calcium excretion
- plasma parathormone (PTH) and Vitamin D concentrations

which can facilitate the diagnosis of

- osteomalacia and rickets
- renal osteodystrophy
- Paget's disease
- hyperparathyroidism (primary, secondary and 'tertiary')
- hypoparathyroidism
- thyroid bone disease

Glucose homeostasis. It is essential that you know normal values for:

- fasting plasma glucose and insulin concentrations
- glucose concentrations during the oral glucose tolerance test (OGTT: see Figure 3.6)

Besides diabetes mellitus (types I and II), the following diagnoses can form the basis of data interpretation questions involving glucose metabolism:

- insulinomas and glucagonomas
- renal glycosuria
- acromegaly
- thyrotoxicosis

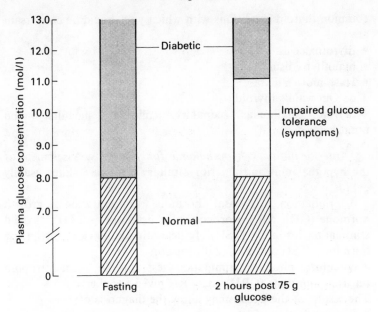

Figure 3.6. Criteria for diagnosis of diabetes and impaired glucose tolerance on the basis of the 75 gram oral glucose tolerance test. If subjects with impaired glucose tolerance do not have symptoms of diabetes, they must also have a plasma glucose concentration greater than 11.0 mmol/l at 30, 60 or 90 minutes post-ingestion.

- post-gastrectomy 'dumping'
- glycogen storage diseases

Other less commonly quoted tests of glucose homeostasis with which it pays to be familiar include:

- intravenous glucose tolerance test (IVGTT)
- fish insulin suppression test

Thyroid function tests. The following assessments of thyroid status commonly appear in data interpretation questions:

- basal total and free triiodothyronine (T3)
- basal total and free thyroxine (T4)
- free thyroxine index (FT4I) which is less commonly quoted with free hormone assays now widely available
- basal thyroid stimulating hormone (TSH)
- thyrotropin releasing hormone (TRH) test

The above tests are altered by pregnancy, drugs and old age, and their results may be accompanied by thyroid antibody titres. The

common thyroid conditions with which you should be conversant are:
• thyrotoxicosis
• hypothyroidism
• Hashimoto's disease
• de Quervain's thyroiditis
• thyroid carcinomas (papillary, follicular, medullary and anaplastic)

Anterior pituitary/hypothalamic function tests. Assessment of the hypothalamus and anterior pituitary in disease states usually entails:
• determination of basal hormone concentrations: growth hormone (GH), adrenocorticotrophic hormone (ACTH), thyroid stimulating hormone (TSH), follicle stimulating and luteinizing hormones (FSH and LH) and prolactin
• combined pituitary stimulation test (insulin, gonadotrophin releasing hormone (GRH) and TRH given together)
The results of these tests may allow the diagnosis of:
• Simmonds' disease
• Sheehan's syndrome
• acromegaly
• prolactinoma

Adrenal function. Adrenal function (cortical and medullary) can be assessed through:
• midnight and 9.00 a.m. plasma cortisol concentrations
• 24-hour urinary free cortisol excretion
• basal plasma ACTH concentration
• dexamethasone suppression test
• metyrapone test
• short and long tetracosactrin tests
• urinary vanillyl mandelic acid (VMA) levels
• plasma catecholamine concentrations (adrenaline and noradrenaline)
The adrenal conditions most frequently encountered in the data interpretation section of the examination are:
• Cushing's disease/syndrome
• Addison's disease
• Conn's syndrome
• adrenogenital syndrome
• phaeochromocytoma

Others. Disorders such as carcinoid syndrome, the porphyrias, Zollinger-Ellison syndrome and the multiple endocrine adenomatoses (Wermer's and Sipple's syndromes) can appear in the data interpretation section. Often the differential diagnosis of a symptom (thirst), a sign (gynaecomastia) or single test result (hypercalcaemia) is at the heart of the question.

Haematology

Full blood count. The full blood count, including the differential white count, platelet count, reticulocyte count and film appearances, can appear in a wide range of data interpretation questions. However, the haematological abnormalities in which it is of prime importance are:
• anaemia (including haemoglobinopathies, sideroblastic anaemia, lead poisoning, haemolytic anaemia, megaloblastic anaemia)
• polycythaemia (relative and absolute)
• leukaemia (acute and chronic) and leucopenia
• thrombocythaemia and thrombocytopenia
• leucoerythroblastic blood picture
• post-transfusion
• post-splenectomy
• hereditary spherocytosis/elliptocytosis

Coagulation/haemostasis. The following data can be presented for analysis (see Figure 3.7):
• prothrombin time (PT)
• kaolin-cephalin coagulation time (KCCT)
• thrombin time (TT)
• bleeding time
• fibrinogen and fibrinogen degradation product (FDP) concentrations
• factor VIII procoagulant and factor VIII – related antigen activities
• Hess test
• platelet aggregation studies (using adenosine diphosphate, collagen and ristocetin)
Typical haematological diagnoses which might be expected from combinations of the above investigations include:
• haemophilia A and B

- von Willebrand's disease
- disseminated intravascular coagulation (DIC)

Others. The range of more specialized haematological tests is large, but useful data may be derived from:
- haemoglobin electrophoresis
- neutrophil alkaline phosphatase (NAP) score
- presence of Philadelphia chromosome
- serum iron/total iron binding capacity (TIBC)/ferritin/folate/ vitamin B_{12} and red cell folate concentrations
- Schilling and Dicopac tests for Vitamin B_{12} deficiency
- serum immunoglobulin concentrations and electrophoresis
- Coombs' test (direct and indirect)
- Ham's test for paroxysmal nocturnal haemoglobinuria
- Donath-Landsteiner test for paroxysmal cold haemoglobinuria

Others

Rheumatology. The diagnosis of diseases such as systemic lupus erythematosus (SLE) and rheumatoid arthritis is based on both

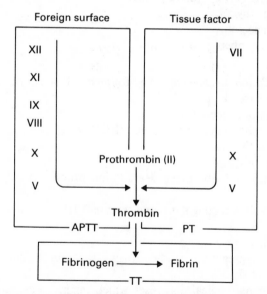

Figure 3.7. Schematic diagram of blood coagulation showing the factors involved in determination of the prothrombin time (PT), activated partial thromboplastin time (APTT–analogous to the KCCT) and thrombin time (TT).

clinical and laboratory findings. Data such as auto-antibody titres, percentage DNA binding and serum complement levels may appear in the examination.

Immunology. Immunological data can appear in questions relating to disease affecting a range of systems from renal medicine (Goodpasture's syndrome and Berger's disease) to gastro-enterology (primary biliary cirrhosis and coeliac disease).

Infectious diseases and tropical medicine. Data interpretation questions are often concerned with patients who have been overseas or who are immigrants to this country. It pays to bear in mind the common diseases affecting this type of patient:
• tuberculosis
• amoebiasis
• malaria
• typhoid

Pharmacology. The drugs a patient is taking commonly influence or cause abnormalities in laboratory data and special tests. Examples of this are:
• antibiotics affecting bioassays for serum folate and B_{12} concentrations
• oral contraceptives influencing thyroid function test results
• anti-tuberculous drugs causing sideroblastic anaemia
• anti-thyroid drugs causing pancytopenia

Trial examination questions

1 A 23-year-old-male, being treated with 'pulsed' methylprednisolone for systemic lupus erythematosus, becomes febrile. On examination there is neck stiffness and marked photophobia. A lumbar puncture is performed. The opening pressure is 280 mmH$_2$O. CSF findings:

Red cells	355/mm^3
White cells	45/mm^3
Protein concentration	0.59 g/l
Glucose concentration	1.9 mmol/l
(plasma glucose concentration	4.2 mmol/l)

Gram and Ziehl-Neelsen stains show no organisms.

Question: What is the diagnosis?
Question: What test would confirm the diagnosis?
Question: What is the treatment?

2 A 45-year-old man was referred from a dermatologist. He had developed an itchy, blistering, erythematous rash which, on biopsy evidence, was diagnosed as 'toxic epidermal necrolysis'. The patient had lost three stone in weight over the previous six months and was found to have a fasting plasma glucose concentration of 13.8 mmol/l.
Question: What is the diagnosis?

3 E.C.G. No. 1

Question: What abnormalities are present?
Question: What immediate management is required?

4 A 68-year-old woman complains of lassitude and weakness. She is noted to be mildly icteric. A full blood count reveals:

Haemoglobin	7.0 g/dl
White cell count	$32.0 \times 10^9/l$
Differential:	92% lymphocytes
	7% neutrophils
	1% monocytes
Mean corpuscular volume	104 fl
Platelet count	$300 \times 10^9/l$

Film comment: polychromasia.

Question: What is the primary diagnosis?
Question: What other condition is evident and what single test would confirm its presence?
Question: What is the treatment?

5 A 14-year-old girl was referred because her G.P. had heard a systolic murmur during a routine physical examination. Results of cardiac catheterization:

	Pressure (mmHg)
Right atrium	5
Right ventricle	20/5
Pulmonary artery	20/9
Pulmonary capillary wedge	8
Left ventricle (high)	145/2
Left ventricle (body)	185/2
After a Valsalva manoeuvre:	
Left ventricle (high)	140/2
Left ventricle (body)	180/2

Question: What is the diagnosis?

6 A boy aged 15 years presents with marked jaundice. He has recently been tired and performing poorly at school, and was sent home the day before admission because of uncontrollable vomiting. He has hepatosplenomegaly.

Haemoglobin concentration	8.0 g/dl
Mean corpuscular volume	110 fl

Reticulocyte count   30%

Plasma concentrations:

sodium	129 mmol/l
potassium	6.1 mmol/l
urea	13.2 mmol/l
creatinine	490 μmol/l
bicarbonate	17 mmol/l

Question: With what condition has he presented acutely?
Question: Suggest an underlying diagnosis and a simple investigation which would confirm it.

·7 A girl of 16 years complains of dyspnoea and simple spirometry is performed:

FEV_1	0.74 litres
FVC	0.87 litres

Arterial blood gases:

$Pa\text{CO}_2$	5.8 kPa
$Pa\text{O}_2$	8.9 kPa
pH	7.30

The houseman administers a drug intravenously and spirometry is repeated:

FEV_1	2.04 litres
FVC	2.40 litres

Question: What drug has been given?
Question: What is the diagnosis?

8 A 42-year-old woman presents with weight loss and malaise. Some months previously she was complaining of mouth ulceration.

Haemoglobin concentration	7.8 g/dl
Mean cellular volume	90 fl

Film comment: acanthocytes, target cells,
   macrocytosis and microcytosis present.
   Howell-Jolly bodies seen.

Question: What is the most likely diagnosis?
Question: The result of which single investigation will confirm the diagnosis?

9 A 35-year-old woman is admitted for investigation of polyuria and polydipsia.

Plasma concentrations:

sodium	144 mmol/l
potassium	3.8 mmol/l
bicarbonate	26 mmol/l
urea	6.8 mmol/l
glucose	4.8 mmol/l
Urine volume	6.5 l/day
Body weight	63.2 kg

She was given chlorpropamide 500 mg by mouth and after 24 hours:

Urine volume	3.8 l/day
Body weight	64.9 kg

Question: What is the diagnosis?

10 An asymptomatic 24-year-old medical student is recruited as a normal volunteer to a drug trial. A biochemical and haematological 'screen' was performed as part of the protocol:

Haemoglobin concentration	14.5 g/dl
White cell count	$6.8 \times 10^9/l$
differential normal	
Platelet count	$195 \times 10^9/l$
Mean corpuscular volume	85 fl
Mean corpuscular haemoglobin concentration	32 g/dl
Reticulocyte count	1.0%

Plasma concentrations:

sodium	139 mmol/l
potassium	4.1 mmol/l
bicarbonate	23 mmol/l
urea	4.2 mmol/l
glucose	3.8 mmol/l

Serum concentrations:

bilirubin	31 μmol/l
aspartate aminotransferase	25 iU/l
alkaline phosphatase	110 iU/l
total protein	73 g/l
albumin	39 g/l
calcium	2.42 mmol/l

Question: What is the diagnosis?

Question : What single test would confirm the diagnosis?

Answers

1 A diagnosis of *cryptococcal meningitis* best fits the data. An *Indian ink stain* will visually reveal the organism in the CSF, although the presence of *cryptococcal antigens* in the CSF at a significant titre is an indication for antifungal therapy. Intravenous *amphotericin B* is conventionally recommended but *flucytosine* is an alternative. *Ketoconazole* may also be of use.

2 The dermatological findings, weight loss and hyperglycaemia all indicate the presence of a *glucagonoma*.

3 The E.C.G. shows evidence of an *acute anterior myocardial infarction* as well as *right bundle branch block* and *right axis deviation*. This is bifascicular block which, in the presence of anterior infarction, is an indication for the *insertion of a pacing wire*.

4 This woman has *chronic lymphocytic leukaemia* complicated by an *autoimmune haemolytic anaemia*. A *Coombs' test* would confirm the presence of the latter condition. *Chlorambucil* is usually used to treat the leukaemia and *corticosteroids* the haemolytic anaemia.

5 The presence of a pressure 'gradient' within the left ventricle indicates a subvalvular obstruction. After the Valsalva manoeuvre, the gradient does not increase which makes the diagnosis of hypertrophic obstructive cardiomyopathy unlikely. A *subvalvar fibrous stenosis or diaphragm* best fits the data.

6 This boy has presented with *haemolytic-uraemic syndrome*. The non-specific prodrome and hepatosplenomegaly suggest a viral infection such as *infectious mononucleosis* and a *Paul-Bunnell test* would be indicated.

7 The administration of *tensilon* to a patient with *myasthenia gravis* would explain the change in spirometry which is not an obstructive picture either before or after the drug is given. The arterial blood gases are consistent with acute-on-chronic respiratory failure.

8 The mouth ulcers, anaemia, dimorphic blood film with evidence of hyposplenism support of diagnosis of *coeliac disease* best diagnosed by the presence of subtotal villous atrophy on *jejunal biopsy*.

9 Chloropropamide stimulates release of ADH from the pituitary and potentiates its action 'on the renal tubule. The data are therefore consistent with a diagnosis of *pituitary diabetes insipidus*.

10 The mild hyperbilirubinaemia suggests *Gilbert's syndrome* which is conventionally diagnosed by an increase in the serum bilirubin concentration with *prolonged fasting* (24 hours).

Chapter 4
The Long Case

What to expect

The long case is normally the first part of the clinical examination. You will be allowed an hour to take a history, perform a full physical examination and collect your thoughts. You will then spend 20 minutes with a pair of examiners who will question you about the case, and you must expect to be taken back to the patient to demonstrate any important physical signs.

Long-case patients should, in theory, be able to provide an adequate history and have enough physical signs to enable the candidate to demonstrate his ability in managing a reasonably complex clinical problem. In practice, you may be faced with a patient who is not a fluent historian and proves difficult to examine, or find that the patient has a surprisingly straightforward diagnosis with little in the way of signs. There are no definite criteria by which patients are selected for this section of the examination.

The examiners may question you about aspects of the history, the interpretation of relevant physical signs and lines of investigation and treatment. Because you have time to obtain a considerable amount of information from the patient, the long case is quite different from the grey cases in the written paper. Moreover, if there is no clear-cut diagnosis, you will usually have the opportunity to discuss the differential diagnosis in detail.

General preparation

The best preparation for the long case is to clerk patients on the wards and in outpatients within a strict 60 minutes. This would include deciding on a policy of management. It is also important to have someone criticize your appraisal of the case and to ask you questions arising from it. Your consultants, senior registrars and registrars will usually be prepared to do this.

In a busy medical job, it is easy to take short cuts when assessing a patient. In the lead-up to the clinical examination, it is advisable to adopt a medical student approach: full history, including

51

comprehensive social and family histories, details of past drug therapy and a thorough physical examination of all systems including the musculoskeletal system and skin.

It is *de rigeur* to make detailed and legible notes as you go. When facing the examiners, trying to find and decipher relevant information can be unnerving if your notes are in a mess. A summary of the case is a useful way of focusing your attention on the main points, starting with the patient's name, age, address and occupation, and progressing to your overall conclusions.

It may be tempting to use only straightforward, co-operative patients in your preparations for the long case. However, having to cope with a difficult patient can prove valuable practice, especially if there is a language barrier confounding your attempts at taking a history or a severe physical disability which interferes with examination.

During the examination

Although ophthalmoscopes, sphygmomanometers and a neurological tray should be provided, most candidates prefer to bring their own equipment to the exam including:
* stethoscope (essential)
* ophthalmoscope (with fresh batteries)
* neurological pins (red and white heads)
* orange sticks
* cotton wool
* torch (also with fresh batteries)
* tongue depressors
* tendon hammer and tuning fork (usually provided and in good order)
* tape measure

These items can be carried in suit pockets or a handbag and may be useful for the short cases as well. Needless to say, you should bring at least two pens and a few sheets of paper, though lined writing paper and a backing board are provided.

At this point, it should be said that your appearance is important. Well-dressed and well-groomed candidates, whether rightly or wrongly, are bound to be viewed more favourably by the examiners. Wearing a white shirt and a sober tie, smelling neutral and shaving off your beard are recommended.

You will be introduced to your patient by an invigilator or examiner. A warm smile and handshake can be difficult to muster in the tension of the moment but may ensure the patient's co-operation from the start. It is sometimes helpful to explain that you are nervous, and to warn that you might have to cut the patients' answers short because of the limited time available to you.

As a rough guide, you should allow 15 minutes for the history which can then continue whilst you are examining the patient. Details of the patients' social circumstances should *always* be asked for and can provide a good lead-in to the rest of the history if you start with this line of questioning. Remember to take complete details of the occupations the patient has had (exposure to asbestos might, for example, have occurred years previously) and to ask specifically how the patient's day-to-day activities are affected by the illness(es). Candidates have failed the examination because they neglected to go into this important area in sufficient detail.

Your approach to history-taking will be primarily influenced by the efficiency and accuracy with which your patient answers questions. You may be lucky enough to be given someone who can tell you his or her diagnosis and treatment, and even the names of the investigations they have undergone. On the other hand, the patient may find it hard keeping to the point. If you are experiencing difficulty in obtaining a good history, it is sometimes worth asking the patient in what his or her doctors (and even the examiners before you arrived) have been most interested.

During physical examination, further clues as to the patient's history may emerge – scars, murmurs, joint deformities and the like can be unexpected findings on the basis of the initial history and the background to these signs should be pursued as you proceed. Even if you are reasonably happy with the history you have obtained, it is worth asking the patient if there is anything you might have missed.

Candidates are often advised to examine the system most relevant to the history first. However, this is important only when you have left yourself insufficient time to perform a complete examination. Otherwise, each system should be appraised fully, including lying and standing blood pressure measurements, a methodical assessment of all groups of lymph nodes, tests of a patient's visual acuity (even if this simply means reading from a newspaper) and other aspects of physical examination which are often left out when patients are seen outside the artificial setting of an exam. You may find, for example, that an elderly patient with chronic granulocytic leukaemia proves to have very poor visual acuity, something which restricts his life a great deal but is not the reason for his presence in hospital.

There are a large number of physical signs which are outside the range of routine examination but which you might be expected to elicit. If, for example, you find the pulse to be collapsing in nature, then the presence of the murmur of aortic incompetence (the 'cardinal sign') confirms the diagnosis. The examiners will be impressed if you have sought and perhaps found Corrigan's, Quinke's and Duroziez's signs.

Again, it is advisable to note down your findings, normal as well as abnormal, system by system. Don't forget to look in the sputum pot if one is present, or to test the patient's urine. Help the patient to dress himself after you have finished your examination, and thank him.

In the final five or ten minutes:
(i) Underline your positive physical findings. This will make them easier to find if the examiners ask for them specifically.
(ii) Write down your diagnosis (with causes), differential diagnosis, relevant investigations, treatment and prognosis.
(iii) Formulate a summary of the case. This should consist of one or two sentences encapsulating the significant aspects of the history and the main physical findings.
(iv) Think of the sorts of questions an examiner would ask you about the case and consider your answers carefully.

During your time with the examiners, you will be called in to present the case (or aspects of it) and then you will be questioned about it. Clearly, a good presentation can prepare the way for a straightforward discussion, whilst a poor presentation means that the candidate will have to do very well during question-time to pass.

When giving the history, it is wise to refer to your notes but you should not bury your head in them and hide. The examiners may interrupt you at any time and it is folly to show annoyance when this happens. Answer what is asked and then return to the presentation. It is very likely that you will be asked specific questions about the history and examination findings and you should be prepared for this. Silence is noisy and obviously doesn't score marks – if you are asked something you cannot answer, say so and move on to the next question.

As in any exam in which you are not limited to a brief answer, there may be a temptation to 'waffle'. Keep your responses as succinct and informative as possible, avoiding abbreviations, vague terms and tangential arguments. The examiners may nod their heads and smile but this does not necessarily mean that you are doing well. A humble but entertaining approach can improve your marks on its own.

A proportion of long cases are 'grey' and thus if you fail to come up with a convincing diagnosis this will not necessarily ruin your changes of passing. The examiners may be more interested in the way you approach management of such a case than an elaborate differential diagnosis.

There is no one system for assessing the long case but the following is commonly adopted:

History

1 Presenting complaint: in the patient's own words.
2 History of the presenting complaint: in chronological order and detailed.
3 Past medical history: again detailed, including all operations and hospital admissions.
4 Family history: a 'family tree' is a useful way of organizing this information.
5 Drug history: present treatment and past drug regimes. Do not forget 'over the counter' medicines such as aspirin.
6 Social and economic circumstances: VERY IMPORTANT. Includes details of social drug use (alcohol, cigarettes and others), financial situation, domestic tensions and practical problems encountered by the patient as a result of disease.
7 Systemic review: thorough. Can unearth significant past medical history that the patient had forgotten.

Examination

Examination of the cardiovascular system
(See Figure 4.1)

1 General observation: for features such as dyspnoea, median sternotomy scar, mitral facies.
2 Hands: cyanosis, clubbing (infective endocarditis, cyanotic con-

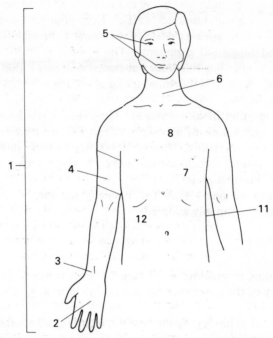

Figure 4.1. A suggested scheme for cardiovascular examination. For a full explanation of the numbered progression, see text.

genital heart disease, arteriovenous fistulae), splinter haemorrhages, sweating, pallid palmar creases, warmth/cold.

3 Radial pulse: rate, rhythm, character. Feel both radials simultaneously. Feel right radial with the right femoral pulse for radio-femoral delay.

4 Blood pressure: lying and standing. If raised, remember to check the fundi.

5 Sclerae and buccal mucosa: cyanosis, pallor, jaundice.

6 Neck: Corrigan's sign, carotid pulse, jugular venous pressure (JVP). Check the wave form of the JVP:

• prominent 'a' wave: pulmonary hypertension, pulmonary stenosis, tricuspid stenosis

• prominent 'v' wave: tricuspid incompetence

• cannon waves: not strictly 'a' waves

7 Apex beat: lowest and outermost point at which the cardiac impulse is palpable. It can be sustained (aortic stenosis, hypertension), tapping (mitral stenosis), heaving (dilated ventricle).

8 Right ventricular heave: indicates pulmonary hypertension if pulmonary stenosis is absent. A 'double kick' suggests left atrial enlargement due to mitral incompetence.

9 Thrills: mitral area and axilla, aortic area and neck, pulmonary and tricuspid areas.

10 Auscultation: time auscultation with thumb or first finger on the carotid pulse (the pulse is equivalent to the first heart sound). Start with bell over the mitral area for mitral stenosis (low pitched) and then use diaphragm for this and all other areas. DO NOT FORGET to lie the patient on his left side for mitral stenosis, and to sit the patient forward and ask him to exhale to accentuate aortic incompetence.

11 Lung bases and sacral area: for basal crackles and oedema respectively.

12 Liver: for enlargement, tenderness, pulsatility (suggesting tricuspid incompetence).

13 Ankles: for oedema.

14 Peripheral pulses.

After you have finished the examination, you should be in a position to decide:

(a) which basic pathological abnormality or abnormalities are present (e.g. valvular heart disease, cardiomyopathy, congenital heart disease, pericarditis).

(b) what functional effect these abnormalities have had (e.g. left and/or right heart failure, arrhythmias, cyanosis pulmonary hypertension, endocarditis).

(c) whether there are any additional physical signs which confirm your cardinal findings (e.g. if there is aortic incompetence: Corrigan's sign, waterhammer pulse, Duroziez's sign, Quinke's sign, pistol-shot femorals).

Examination of the respiratory system
(See Figure 4.2)

1 General observation: note the use of accessory muscles of respiration and the presence of dyspnoea, wheeze, stridor, chest deformities and scars. Look for the sputum pot.

2 Hands: cyanosis, clubbing (chronic pulmonary suppuration, intrathoracic malignancy, fibrosing alveolitis), signs of carbon dioxide retention (warm hands, dilated veins, flapping tremor).

3 Radial pulse: bounding (hypercapnia), paradox.

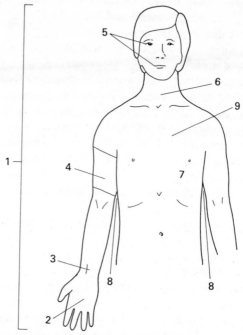

Figure 4.2. A suggested scheme for examination of the respiratory system. For a full explanation of the numbered progression, see text.

4 Blood pressure: paradox.
5 Eyes: pupils and fundi (hypercapnia).
  Mouth: central cyanosis.
6 Neck: jugular venous pressure (superior vena caval obstruction), lymph nodes, trachea (displacement, tracheostomy scar).
7 Apex beat: displacement.
8 Axillae: lymph nodes.
9 Chest examination:
(i) Inspection: lie the patient flat and observe the rise and fall of the chest from the end of the bed – this is a sensitive way of observing the mechanics of breathing.
(ii) Palpation: assess expansion, test for tactile fremitus.
(iii) Percussion: do not forget the apices. Compare sides and try, as with auscultation, to relate your findings to the surface markings of the lungs. Effective percussion will not disturb the patient and will make abnormalities evident to an observer standing nearby. It may

be necessary to percuss for the level and movement of the diaphragm.

(vi) Auscultation: with the patient breathing through his open mouth. Report on presence and timing of crackles, rubs and wheezes. Again, compare sides and assess vocal resonance.

In the long case you may be asked how to assess the patient's respiratory function without the aid of technology. Some useful indicators are:

• the history: e.g. can the patient walk up a flight of stairs without stopping?

• maximal chest expansion: if less than two inches (5 cm) airflow obstruction is likely.

• forced expiration time: if greater than four seconds, airflow obstruction is again likely.

• blowing out a lighted match: hold a match six inches away from the patient's open mouth. If, during forced expiration, the flame does not flicker, the peak flow is usually less than 60 litres/minute. If the flame flickers but does not go out, the peak flow is of the order of 60–100 litres/minute. If the flame goes out, the peak flow is at least 100 litres/minute.

• clinical assessment of arterial blood gases: cyanosis indicates hypoxia but this also depends on the haemoglobin concentration. Peripheral and central signs of hypercapnia may be present.

After you have finished your examination, decide:

(a) whether there is any evidence of long-standing chest disease (chronic airways obstruction, tuberculosis and bronchiectasis for example).

(b) whether there are abnormalities present which suggest an acute problem (pneumonia, pneumothorax and asthma for example).

(c) what sequelae have resulted from (a) and (b) (such as cor pulmonale and restricted exercise tolerance).

Examination of the nervous system

1 General observation: including the face (Sturge-Weber syndrome, tuberose sclerosis), the skin (neurofibromatosis, the scars of syringomyelia), the legs (peroneal muscle atrophy) – often the diagnosis is made on observation alone. Always establish whether the patient is left or right handed.

2 Higher centres: orientation (time, place, person), mood, memory (short and long term), intellect (abstract thought, arithmetic ability,

general knowledge), speech (dysphasia, dysarthria, dysphonia). Generally-accepted tests (serial 7's, Babcock sentences and so on) are best used.

3 Cranial nerves:

I: if smell bottles are provided, a quick assessment is easy.

II: acuity can be assessed in the absence of a Snellen chart by the patient's ability to read newsprint with each eye in turn. Use neurological pins for visual field assessment and test specifically for central scotomata. Fundoscopy should *always* be performed.

II, III: pupillary relexes to light *and* accommodation.

III, IV, VI: test full range of movements noting diplopia and nystagmus.

V: the corneal reflexes are often forgotten, as is the jaw jerk.

VII: weakness should always be classified as either upper or lower motor neurone.

VIII: Rinne's and Weber's tests: remember which is which.

IX: gag reflex and a chance to inspect the oropharynx.

X: assess swallowing.

XI: sternomastoid and trapezius.

XII: fasciculation of the tongue is probably over-diagnosed.

4 The limbs and trunk:

(i) Inspection: for wasting, fasciculation, contractures, abnormal movement (tremor, chorea, athetosis etc.).

(ii) Palpation: for muscle bulk and tenderness.

(iii) Tone: assess with distraction if indicated.

(iv) Power: if you use the MRC scale, know what the grades mean. 'Mild', 'moderate' or 'severe' weakness is usually an adequate assessment of loss of power.

(v) Reflexes: do not forget the abdominals. Be wary about referring to the plantar responses as 'equivocal'. Use reinforcement if the reflexes are unobtainable.

(vi) Sensation: all modalities. Try to compare any abnormalities with dermatome distribution.

(vii) Co-ordination: standard tests (such as finger-nose and heel-shin) are best used. Assessment of *gait* is very important and often forgotten, as is Romberg's test.

5 Additional tests (such as handwriting, assessment of spatial orientation and glabellar tap) may be required.

After you have finished your examination, you should decide:

(a) where, on the basis of the signs you have found, the anatomical lesion(s) is/are located.

(b) what pathological diagnosis or diagnoses are probable on the basis of the history and examination.

(c) which investigations you would consider requesting to confirm your diagnosis.

Examination of the gastrointestinal system
(See Figure 4.3)

For convenience, this will include the genito-urinary system.

1 General observation: for features such as abdominal distension, spider naevi, pyoderma gangrenosum, erythema nodosum, telangiectasia, oedema, bruising.

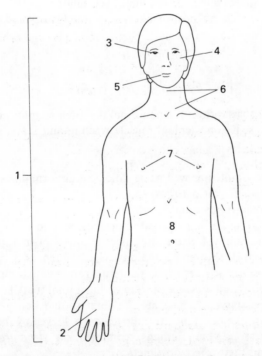

Figure 4.3. A suggested scheme for gastrointestinal examination. For a full explanation of the numbered progression, see text.

2 Hands: clubbing, liver nails, Dupuytren's contractures, wasting, flapping tremor, palmar erythema.

3 Sclerae: for pallor and jaundice.

4 Parotid glands: for enlargement.

5 Buccal mucosa and tongue: foetor, angular stomatitis, glossitis.

6 Left supraclavicular fossa and axillae: for lymph node enlargement.

7 Breasts: for gynaecomastia.

8 Abdomen:

(i) Inspection: with the patient lying flat, look for scars, striae, hair distribution, obvious swellings, movement (with respiration, peristalsis, pulsation), dilated veins.

(ii) Palpation: for the liver, spleen, kidneys, bladder, aorta, herniae, inguinal lymph nodes, genitalia.

(iii) Percussion: over organs and palpable masses, and for ascites.

(iv) Auscultation: arterial bruits and bowel sounds.

When you have completed your examination:

(a) consider your findings in rough order of significance (e.g. a very large spleen ahead of minimal liver enlargement).

(b) decide which diagnosis is likely from the history and examination.

Examination of the musculoskeletal system

1 General observation: for abnormalities such as joint deformity, contractures, leg shortening, muscle wasting and scars. Compare sides.

2 Inspection:

(i) Gait: locomotor as well as neurological abnormalities give rise to characteristic gait patterns.

(ii) Posture: kyphosis and/or scoliosis.

(iii) Joints, muscles and related structures: should include assessment of the range of active movement at any abnormal joint, and measurement of shortening and limb circumferences if indicated.

3 Palpation: for joint swelling, tenderness and temperature, as well as for crepitus and presence of fluid within a joint (patella tap). The range of passive movement at each joint should be assessed and compared to the range of active movement achieved by the patient. When assessing your findings, comment on *structural* abnormalities and their effect on *function*.

Typical examination material

Patients with the following diagnoses often appear as long cases in the exam:

Cardiology

Ischaemic heart disease: patients with this diagnosis will usually have a complication (e.g. left ventricular aneurysm).

Valvular heart disease: usually mitral or aortic. A history of rheumatic fever should be sought: with aortic incompetence in a young person, the seronegative arthritides must be considered.

Cardiomyopathies: will usually be of the dilated variety. Hypertrophic obstructive cardiomyopathy (HOCM) is very difficult to diagnose clinically.

Congenital heart disease: acyanotic and cyanotic. Rare but appear in the exam because of their signs.

Respiratory medicine

Chronic airflow obstruction: ask specifically about a history of cough with sputum production (chronic bronchitis). Emphysema is, strictly speaking, a pathological diagnosis.

Carcinoma of the bronchus: its possible presentations are legion (including neuromuscular, endocrine and dermatological) and you should be aware of these; the main histological types of tumour, and modern approaches to treatment (e.g. the value of chemotherapy in oat cell carcinoma).

Fibrosing alveolitis: is a rare disease but its clinical signs (including clubbing and showers of fine, end-inspiratory crackles on auscultation), investigation and management provide a lot to talk about.

Old tuberculosis: is a good source of physical signs. The patient may have had such procedures as pneumonectomy, lobectomy and formation of an artificial pneumothorax which can make assessment more difficult.

Pneumoconioses: are uncommon in the exam but, needless to say, a full occupational history is mandatory.

Asthma: if the patient has had this condition chronically, complications of steroid therapy may be in evidence.

Neurology

Multiple sclerosis: always consider this in patients with apparently unrelated physical signs and a vague history.

Motor neuron disease: it is wise to know the various types and what abnormalities are expected on relevant investigations (e.g. electromyography).

Cerebrovascular disease: if there is evidence of a stroke, examine the cardiovascular system carefully.

Parkinson's disease: causes and treatment are favourite discussion points.

Peripheral neuropathy: there is usually evidence of pathology in other systems (the patient may, for example, have diabetes, alcoholic liver disease or a malignancy).

Gastroenterology

Chronic liver disease: usually easy to identify from the physical signs. The history may well give the cause (e.g. alcohol, viral, Wilson's disease).

Inflammatory bowel disease: these patients may have few signs but their management can provide a lot for discussion.

Malabsorption: including coeliac disease and post-gastrectomy. These cases will often lead on to questions about the investigation of malabsorption.

Gastrointestinal malignancies: although considered 'surgical' by many, these can still appear as long cases in the exam.

Haematology

Chronic leukaemias: often included because of their striking physical signs. Non-leukaemic myeloproliferative disorders also appear.

Rheumatology

Collagen vascular diseases: because these are multisystem disorders, they can have a good range of signs. Investigation and treatment are fruitful areas for discussion.

In general, patients who are to spend an hour as examination subjects have to have a degree of 'stamina'. As a general rule, those with chronic diseases usually appear: patients who are acutely unwell are unsuitable.

Chapter 5
The Short Cases

What to expect

In the short case section, candidates can expect to be shown up to ten cases within 20 minutes. One pair of examiners will take the candidate for the first half of the exam before a second pair takes over. This means that each examiner will have five minutes of the candidate's time.

The range of examination material is potentially large but, as discussed below, there are a number of cases which come up with regularity. The extent of the physical examination you will be required to perform is variable, from a 'spot' diagnosis to a detailed assessment of a patient's neurological state. You may be interrupted at any time and asked what you are doing, have found or intend to do next. However, it is more usual for a candidate to be allowed to finish his examination before being questioned.

It is often said that the more short cases one sees, the better the performance, but candidates have passed after examining only two or three patients. Diagnostic complexity and the approach of the examiners may well have more bearing on how much time you spend with a particular case than your own clinical ability.

General preparation

Hospital wards and outpatient clinics are rich sources of potential short cases. Your registrars and consultants are usually willing to oversee your examination and question you about your findings. It is sometimes better to be examined by someone unpleasant as this can sharpen your presentation considerably.

Unlike the long case, your examination technique will be under close scrutiny. It is therefore essential that you can examine any short case within three minutes in a confident and competent manner. This includes getting into the habit of introducing yourself, shaking hands, positioning the patient so that he is comfortable and easy to examine and establishing whether any of the manoeuvres you are about to perform might induce pain. It is self-evident that to hurt a patient during the exam will not help your chances of passing.

After sufficient practice on short cases, you should be able to perform a complete examination and start to marshal your thoughts *whilst* examining. This entails both organizing your findings and arriving at a diagnosis: you may well be asked about nothing more.

The way you answer questions will also need practice under exam conditions. Always *answer the question*: if you are asked for the abnormal physical signs, simply list them. If you are asked for a diagnosis, give the one you think the most appropriate. You may be able to add, '. . . as evidenced by the following signs . . .', in support of your answer but the examiners may not want any further information. The time-honoured 'do's and don'ts' of clinical examinations still apply:

• hands behind back to avoid gesticulations
• look the examiner in the eyes
• avoid ums and errs, and prefaces such as 'I think' and 'there might have been'
• use 'sir' if you think it appropriate
• avoid long silences even if this means asking for the question to be repeated
• do not confabulate: a simple 'I don't know' may save you from getting into hot water
• say 'thank you' to the patient at the end of the exam.

For most candidates, the development of a good short-case technique will require considerable practice. The more cases you see in the run-up to the exam, the more efficient and assured you will be.

During the examination

You will be introduced to your first pair of examiners and one of them will direct you to the patients. It is important to create a good impression during the first case as this will probably set the tone during the rest of the exam. A practised approach is the best antidote to the nervousness which is inevitably at its peak when you start.

It is dangerous to assume that the patients have been prepared for you. If you think that the patient is not at 45° to the horizontal then reposition him before starting to examine the cardiovascular system. Similarly, if the patient is not adequately exposed this should, with due allowance for the patient's decorum, be seen to before you begin. Whilst preparing the patient, there is often time to look for bedside diagnostic clues – sputum pots, bottles of diabetic squash, a peak-flow meter and so on.

Whilst examining the patient, if you concentrate on the system you have practised your omissions should be few. If you remember during the examination something you should have done earlier, go back and do it at the next opportunity rather than leave it out – it may reveal an important physical sign. Do what you are told – examination of the praecordium does not mean starting with palpation of the radial pulse. If you are unsure exactly what the examiner expects of you, ask him to repeat his instructions.

The examiner's questions are usually delivered within earshot of the patient. It is important to avoid using words that might be taken at face value. A patient with old tuberculosis might well become very upset if you use the word 'cancer' when discussing possible causes for the signs you have elicited.

After each short case, it is common courtesy to thank the patient. Examiners will not be impressed if you leave a patient exposed and uncomfortable, and it is wise to rectify this before moving on to the next case.

Candidates who feel they have done very poorly early on in the short case section often lose heart and their subsequent performance is affected. It is wise to remember that you are in the worst possible position to judge your own performance during the exam and that mistakes are very often retrievable.

Typical examination material

The short case section is the most feared part of the examination. This is probably because candidates believe that any case can be thrown at them and that vague or tangential questions may be asked. This is far from true and the fourteen short cases described below will cover the majority of those you will encounter in the exam. Regardless of what you see, the examiners' questions are virtually always limited to one or more of the following:

- What are your findings?
- What is your diagnosis?
- What other physical signs would you look for?
- What are the causes of . . .?

Short case 1: 'Feel the pulse'

Do as you are told. Do not start an examination of the cardiovascular system. Count the beats over fifteen seconds noting regularity/ir-regularity. Continue feeling the pulse and assess its character. Is it collapsing (aortic incompetence)? Is it slow rising (aortic stenosis)? Then look at the patient for clues. Is he thyrotoxic? There may be atrial fibrillation. Is there evidence of mitral facies? The examination should take no more than about 30–45 seconds.

Question: 'What are your findings?'

Describe the rate, regularity and nature of the pulse without making a diagnosis, e.g. 'The heart rate is 36/minute, regular and of normal character'.

Question: 'What is the cause of this?'

If the heart rate is slow (less than 40 beats/minute) the two diagnoses would be complete heart block and sinus bradycardia. If fast and regular the diagnosis would include sinus tachycardia and a variety of supraventricular tachycardias. If the heart is fast and irregular there is a temptation to say the patient is in atrial fibrillation. Beware, the patient may be in sinus rhythm with multiple atrial and/or ventricular ectopics.

Further questions clearly depend on the foregoing answers. If the pulse is slow the examiner will ask you how you decide which rhythm it is. He may ask the candidate to elicit other signs of complete heart block (variable first heart sound, cannon waves in the neck and an ejection systolic murmur). If the pulse is fast (e.g. atrial fibrillation) the examiner may want a list of causes. It is tempting to suggest the rarest because they have a habit of sticking in the brain. The answer 'pericardial secondaries from carcinoma of the bronchus' will stimulate the examiner's irritable colon. The commonest causes of atrial fibrillation are:

• ischaemic heart disease
• mitral valve disease
• dilated cardiomyopathy
• thyrotoxicosis
• any other form of heart disease

If the patient has a collapsing pulse and both you and the examiner have agreed it is due to aortic incompetence he will ask either,

'What are the causes of aortic incompetence?' (bicuspid aortic valve disease, rheumatic heart disease, dissecting aneurysm and so on), or, more likely, 'What other signs of aortic incompetence would you look for?' (collapsing pulse, waterhammer pulse, Corrigan's sign, Quinke's sign, Duroziez's sign etc.).

If there is time, you may be asked about management. Be prepared to talk about pacemaker insertion and the drug treatment of arrhythmias.

Short case 2: 'Examine the jugular veins'

Despite what cardiologists say, the jugular venous pressure is extremely difficult to examine. The patient MUST be positioned correctly at 45° to the horizontal. Look at the veins using a torch if you have one. This will impress the examiner even if you don't quite know what you are doing but it should throw the architecture of the neck into relief. Two features must be noted:

(i) The height of the jugular venous pressure. It is perfectly permissible to use the external jugular vein if it rises and falls freely. Observe for pulsation of the earlobes; when the pressure is very high this may be the only clue. Ideally, measure the height of the JVP with a ruler as one is often very inaccurate when guessing.

(ii) The waveform. After you have decided the height of the JVP, place your thumb on the carotid artery. A wave in the jugular vein coincident with the carotid pulsation is a 'v' wave and a wave preceding will be an 'a' wave. Beware of cannon waves which are intermittent and not true 'a' waves. Large 'v' waves are due to tricuspid incompetence and at first glance may make the whole neck pulsate, giving the appearance of aortic incompetence.

Question: 'What are your findings?'

Describe the height and waveform of the jugular venous pressure. Do not say 'JVP'

Question: 'What might be the cause of this?'

If there is only a raised venous pressure which you observe to rise and fall with respiration, the causes would be:
• congestive cardiac failure
• renal failure
• other causes of fluid overload

If the venous pressure in the neck is clearly raised but fixed, the cause would be some form of obstruction (e.g. superior vena caval). If there is an obviously abnormal jugular venous pulsation, diagnostic clues will be in prominence of the wave form:

'v' wave – tricuspid incompetence
'v' wave – tricuspid incompetence
'a' wave – pulmonary hypertension
– pulmonary stenosis
– tricuspid stenosis

Question: 'What else would you wish to examine?'

This depends on the answer to the previous question. If, for example, you suspect congestive cardiac failure, a cardiovascular examination would be indicated. Prominent 'v' waves would mean special attention to signs such as liver pulsation and peripheral oedema, while a prominent 'a' wave would require you to look for evidence of right ventricular hypertrophy.

It is possible to be asked the treatment of a raised jugular venous pressure and this clearly depends on the cause.

Short case 3: 'Listen to the heart'

This may form part of a complete examination of the cardiovascular system but, because this takes some time, listening directly to the heart is more commonly requested. There is virtually a fifty per cent chance of getting this short case in the exam.

First feel for the apex beat as this is the mitral area. Put your stethoscope over this area and put your thumb on the carotid artery (the carotid pulsation more or less equals the first heart sound). Use the bell of the stethoscope as this will pick up the low pitched sounds of mitral stenosis. Then turn your stethoscope to the diaphragm and listen over the mitral area, and then the axilla, the tricuspid area, the pulmonary area, the aortic area and the carotids.

Next roll the patient on his left side; this will accentuate mitral stenosis. Finally, sit the patient forward and listen for aortic incompetence during exhalation. If you think there may be mitral stenosis (e.g. if mitral facies are present) sit the patient up and down six times and listen again. As you listen note:
• sounds
• added sounds

• murmurs

in that order.

Question: 'What did you hear?'

It is often difficult to describe your findings unless you stick to a strict order. Take each area in turn, and describe the sounds, added sounds and murmurs. For example, 'The first and second heart sounds were normal and there were no added sounds. In the mitral area I heard a soft, pansystolic murmur which radiated to the axilla and which was compatible with mitral incompetence. In the aortic area I heard a soft decrescendo diastolic murmur which was compatible with aortic incompetence. There were no other murmurs to be heard.'

If the patient is over the age of 40 years, the murmurs which will be heard are most likely to be aortic or mitral. It is very unwise to go into this examination not knowing how to describe the murmurs of aortic stenosis and incompetence, together with the severity of the valvular disease in question.

Mitral stenosis. The closer the murmur to the second sound, the tighter the stenosis. Conversely, if there is a long gap between the second sound and the start of the murmur, the stenosis will be mild (see Figure 5.1).

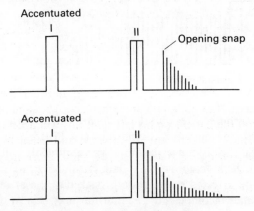

Figure 5.1. Mild (above) and tight (below) mitral stenosis.

Mitral stenosis can also be 'pliable' or 'rigid'. A pliable valve suggests little scarring and may be treatable by a valvotomy. A rigid valve would need to be replaced by a prosthetic valve. Signs of pliability are the presence of an opening snap, late accentuation of the murmur and a loud first heart sound (see Figure 5.2).

Note that the time-honoured idea that late accentuation of the murmur only occurs in sinus rhythm is incorrect. It may occur in atrial fibrillation if the valve is pliable.

Mitral incompetence. The murmur is soft, pansystolic and radiates to the axilla. The first heart sound is usually soft. Signs of severe mitral incompetence are the presence of a pansystolic murmur with a third heart sound and a soft diastolic murmur (see Figure 5.3). When mitral incompetence is severe, tricuspid incompetence may also be present.

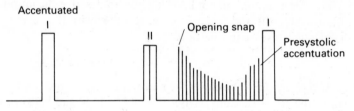

Figure 5.2. Pliable mitral stenosis.

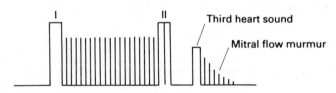

Figure 5.3. Severe mitral incompetence.

Mitral incompetence and the billowing mitral leaflet syndrome. There are three stages in this syndrome (see Figure 5.4). A solitary mid-systolic click is due to the mitral valve suddenly ballooning out during ventricular contraction. A late systolic murmur may also be heard as the affected cusp balloons back into the atrium and the valve becomes incompetent. The murmur may be soft or loud and can be likened, in some cases, to a 'cooing dove' or 'seagull'. It is perhaps best to avoid these expressions in the exam. A pan-systolic murmur results when the mitral cusp becomes detached from its chordae tendinae producing significant mitral incompetence.

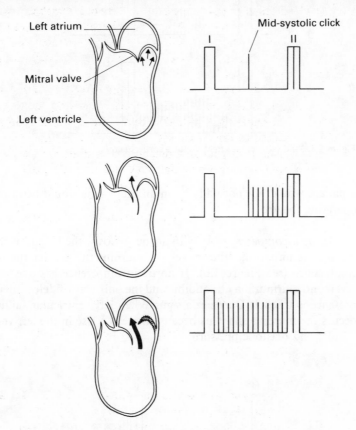

Figure 5.4. Billowing mitral valve leaflet syndrome. This can vary from a mid-systolic click (above), to a late systolic murmur and mid-systolic click (middle), to frank mitral incompetence (below) depending on the stage.

Aortic stenosis. The length of the murmur is everything (see Figure 5.5). A short murmur represents mild aortic stenosis. A long murmur which obliterates the second sound indicates tight aortic stenosis. The murmur of aortic stenosis is harsh, ejection-type and radiates to the carotids. Remember that as left ventricular failure develops, the murmur of tight aortic stenosis gets shorter. But such

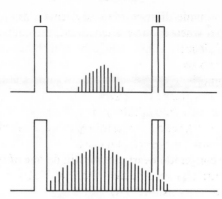

Figure 5.5. Mild (above) and tight (below) aortic stenosis.

a patient would not normally be in an exam – he would be in the operating theatre.

Aortic incompetence. As with aortic stenosis, the length of the murmur is important: the longer the murmur the greater the incompetence (see Figure 5.6). If aortic incompetence is extremely severe, no murmur may be audible and the only way of detecting its presence is to elicit Duroziez's sign. When left ventricular failure occurs the murmur shortens because there is a rise in the left ventricular end diastolic pressure.

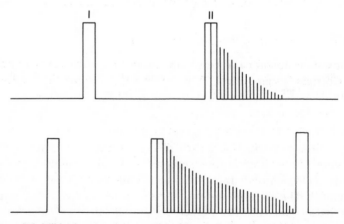

Figure 5.6. Mild (above) and severe (below) aortic incompetence.

A young patient under the age of twenty years is most likely to have congenital heart disease. If he is cyanosed, remember the 't's':
- tetralogy of Fallot
- truncus arteriosus
- tricuspid stenosis
- transposition of the great vessels
- total anomalous venous drainage

These patients will have a systolic murmur but it will not be possible to make an accurate diagnosis clinically.

Acyanotic congenital heart disease will be one of the following:
- atrial or ventricular septal defect (ASD or VSD)
- patent ductus arteriosus (PDA)
- coarctation (*always* feel for radio-femoral delay)
- pulmonary stenosis

If you hear no murmurs, the presence of a large heart and added sounds (third or fourth heart sounds, or a gallop), suggest a dilated cardiomyopathy.

Further questions from the examiners will depend on what you have found. Mitral and aortic valve diseases usually have other signs which you could be asked to elicit, or you might be asked for causes. For acyanotic congenital heart disease, you could be requested to list necessary investigations and outline treatment (e.g. cardiac catheterization for an atrial septal defect followed by surgical closure if the left-to-right shunt is greater than 2:1). The causes of a dilated cardiomyopathy (idiopathic, alcohol, pregnancy and myxoedema) can also serve as subject matter for further questions.

Short case 4: 'Examine this patient's neck'

Look at the neck for a few seconds. Are there any obvious swellings? Is Corrigan's sign evident? Your examination should then concentrate on each of the structures present: arteries, veins, lymph glands, trachea and thyroid.

First examine the patient from behind using the time-honoured technique of asking the patient to drink from a glass of water to allow optimal examination of the thyroid gland. Is it nodular? Is it hard or soft? Then feel for lymph gland enlargement in the anterior, posterior and supraclavicular triangles.

Next come round to the front of the patient and check that the trachea is central. Look at the neck veins (see Short Case 2) and feel the carotid pulses. Percussion for a retrosternal thyroid may also be necessary. Finally take out your stethoscope and listen for bruits over the carotids and thyroid gland.

Question: 'What are your findings?'

Describe the abnormalities without too many negatives. It is sometimes useful to base your answer on the familiar *inspection, palpation, percussion, auscultation* scheme.

Question: 'What other physical signs would you look for?'

This depends on the answer to the previous question. If the thyroid gland is enlarged or there is a thyroidectomy scar, you may be expected to look for signs of hyper- or hypothyroidism. If you find a carotid bruit, look for signs of an old stroke. The previous short case covers findings relating to the jugular veins, whilst if the trachea is deviated you may be asked to examine the chest. If there are enlarged lymph glands, be sure to think of their drainage area (see Figure 5.7). Painless glands would suggest Hodgkin's disease particularly if very large and in a young patient. Painful glands might indicate infection in the appropriate drainage area.

Occasionally the examiner will be looking to the candidate to identify the use of accessory muscles of respiration as a lead-in to an examination of the chest. Rarely, superior vena caval obstruction may appear and chest signs may also be present.

Short case 5: 'Examine the chest'

This is often limited to an examination of the front or the back of the chest. Try to adhere to the scheme outlined in Chapter 4. Some simple guidelines are as follows:

1 if respiratory movements are decreased on one side of the chest, the pathology will be on that side.

2 never forget to check for tracheal deviation and remember to do tactile fremitus as part of palpation: this latter manoeuvre is often forgotten because it is not done routinely outside the setting of the examination.

3 dullness to percussion represents definite pathology though resonance may also be elicited when pathology is present.

4 the examiners will be impressed if you demonstrate the abnor-

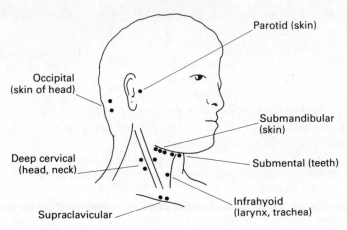

Figure 5.7. The major groups of cervical lymph nodes and their drainage areas.

malities clearly before describing them: the 'stony dull' percussion note of a pleural effusion can be made obvious without inflicting discomfort on the patient.

5 beware of spending too much time on auscultation: if you take twenty seconds or more to convince yourself that you can hear bronchial breathing over one area of the chest wall, the examiners will become bored.

Question: 'What are your findings?'

This should be a straightforward description. You should be careful not to become confused over the anatomical position of the signs you have found (e.g. to say 'left' instead of 'right': see Figure 5.8). If your signs seem inconsistent with a single diagnosis, give the most important and definite signs first. There may be dual pathology present as an explanation for your findings but this will usually be apparent from the examiner's line of questioning.

Question: 'What is the diagnosis?'

The commonest chest cases seen in the examination are:
• chronic airflow obstruction
• pulmonary fibrosis (e.g. old tuberculosis)
• lobectomy/pneumonectomy
• pleural effusion

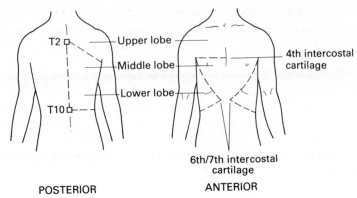

Figure 5.8. Anatomical landmarks which are of use in describing physical signs in the chest.

- consolidation and collapse
- bronchiectasis

Strictly speaking, terms such as 'pleural effusion' and 'fibrosis' are *not* diagnoses but the examiners may not expect you to go any further than this. However, if you have, for example, found a pleural effusion in an elderly, cachectic man with heavily nicotine-stained fingers and enlarged axillary lymph nodes, the examiners would expect you to mention that he may have a malignant effusion secondary to an underlying bronchogenic carcinoma.

Further questions will depend on your findings. If the patient has chronic airflow obstruction, you might be asked how you would assess lung function at the bedside (see Chapter 4). If the patient has had a lobectomy, you might be asked the possible reasons for this. If there is no obvious cause for a pleural effusion, you may be asked how it should be investigated.

Short case 6: 'Examine this patient's abdomen'

This is a common short case but is usually straightforward. Lie the patient flat with his head on a single pillow. Observe the abdomen for a few seconds during which the patient should be instructed to take a deep breath. This manoeuvre can make visible swellings more obvious.

Ask the patient if he has any abdominal tenderness. Palpate and percuss for the liver, spleen and kidneys; this is best done from a kneeling position. Then check for masses, the presence of an aortic aneurysm and examine for herniae. If ascites is likely, test for shifting dullness. Ask the examiner if it is acceptable to examine the genitalia and rectum: it will normally be unnecessary. Finish with auscultation; this is frequently forgotten.

If you are told to examine the gastrointestinal system start with the hands, check the skin for signs of liver failure, and then look at the sclerae for jaundice and anaemia. Palpate for parotid enlargement and examine the mouth and tongue. Feel for supraclavicular lymph node enlargement and check for gynaecomastia.

Proper examination of the main abdominal organs is extremely important:

Liver. With the patient breathing through his mouth, palpate with the forefinger parallel to the liver edge; keep the hand still during inspiration. Start in the right lower quadrant and move upwards. Feel the edge for consistency, regularity, tenderness and pulsatility. Palpate its surface and demonstrate that you cannot get above it. Percuss its lower and upper borders, moving up from below and down from above (i.e. from resonant to dull). Identify the interspace at which the upper border lies and demonstrate the liver span in the mid-clavicular line.

Spleen. As for the liver, start in the right lower quadrant and move up towards the left costal margin. If the spleen is enlarged, try to identify its notch and palpate its surface. Show that you cannot get above it, and percuss from resonant to dull. If indicated, examine the patient in the right lateral position.

Kidneys. Palpate bimanually. Feel their surfaces if possible and demonstrate that you can get above them. They should move with respiration and will normally be resonant to percussion.

Question: 'What are your findings?'

The likeliest abnormalities are an enlarged liver and/or splenomegaly. Polycystic kidneys are an examination favourite and should always be borne in mind if you should find unilateral or bilateral renal masses. Aortic aneurysms rarely appear, whilst other masses (such as a gastric or colonic carcinoma, enlarged gallbladder or inguinal lymphadenopathy) are also uncommonly encountered.

Question: 'What are the causes of your findings?'

The causes of an enlarged liver are many and additional features (such as the presence of pulsatility or an irregular edge) will usually direct you to an appropriate differential diagnosis. As in any short case, to start with a diagnosis such as Gaucher's disease as a cause for apparently isolated hepatomegaly is inviting trouble; give common causes first.

Splenomegaly is conventionally divided into 'massive' (which can extend into the right lower quadrant), 'moderate' and 'mild' (normally just palpable below the costal margin), and a rough classification of causes can be based on this. Again, to mention malaria as your first diagnosis of a moderately enlarged spleen in a well-looking Caucasian may spur the examiner to ask about the changing patterns of chloroquine resistance.

Further questions may suggest that there are signs to be found in other systems (cardiovascular and reticuloendothelial for example). If you have found genito-urinary signs, the examiners may expect you to ask to see a sample of urine.

Short case 7: 'Examine the arms/legs'

In the limbs, the structures present are arteries, veins, nerves, joints, lymph glands and skin. It is easy to miss out an important aspect of the examination unless you have a well-rehearsed system. Always remember to compare sides.

Inspect the limbs quickly for any obvious clues as to the diagnosis (e.g. a swollen joint, black toe or claw hand). If there is no such clue, start with the nervous system (which will take the most time), then proceed to the vasculature, joints, lymph nodes and skin (including the nails).

Some general points are:
• if there are rheumatoid hands (or feet) do not forget to examine for nodules. These may, for example, be hidden underneath a patient's partially rolled up sleeves
• listen for femoral and popliteal bruits if there is peripheral vascular disease in the lower limbs
• do not forget to examine the posterior surfaces of the legs: there may be sensory abnormalities which are not present elsewhere and the heels can be sites of neuropathic ulcers

• in the unlikely event that you are asked to examine a leg with obvious varicose veins, it is wise to know how to perform a Trendelenburg test.

Question: 'What are your findings?'

Peripheral neuropathy (motor and sensory), hemiplegias, diplegias, Parkinsonism and multiple sclerosis are common neurological cases. You must know the signs of ulnar, median and radial nerve palsies, as well as the various causes and distributions of wasting of the small muscles of the hand. Syringomyelia is often brought out for the exam. Marshal your findings as for the long case (see Chapter 4). Because neurological cases are often complex, you will probably not get much beyond this first question and subsequent questions will depend purely on the diagnosis. You might, for example, be asked what other signs of the disease might be found in other parts of the body.

The only major abnormality in the arterial system is narrowing of the arteries. Diabetes is always a possible background problem; occasionally you will be expected to find a popliteal artery aneurysm.

Joint pathology would include osteoarthritis, rheumatoid arthritis, psoriatic arthropathy and gout. Skin rashes become important here as well as a part of the question, 'What other signs would you look for?'

Problems in the venous system are extremely unusual exam cases, being limited to deep venous thrombosis or varicose veins.

Examination of the lymph glands is particularly relevant if the limb is swollen. This may well lead on to the candidate being asked to examine the reticuloendothelial system as a whole.

Short case 8: 'Examine the cranial nerves'

Although you may be asked to examine the cranial nerves as a whole, it is more likely that you will be asked to assess only some of them. The two most likely short cases in this respect are
• examination of the face (cranial nerves V and VII)
• examination of the eyes (cranial nerves II, III, IV and VI)
Examining the eyes is usually performed very badly because there is a lot to do and the candidate can easily forget to examine one cranial nerve altogether.

The eyes. Inspect the eyes for ptosis, jaundice, arcus senilis and anaemia. Check that the patient is not blind: cover each eye in turn and ask him first to count fingers and then to read print. Check the visual fields with pinheads. Inspect both pupils and try to elicit the light and accommodation reflexes bilaterally. Examine the fundi. Test all external ocular muscles: look for nystagmus and ask about diplopia. Beware of the glass eye.

The face. Check all three divisions of the trigeminal nerve with cotton wool: use pinprick to delineate the anaesthetic area. Check the corneal reflexes. The examiners may expect you to complete the examination of the Vth nerve by testing the pterygoids and eliciting the jaw jerk. Turn to the seventh nerve and test for the presence of upper and lower motor neuron lesions. Assessment of taste is usually not required.

Question: 'What are your findings?'

There is likely to be a total or partial palsy of one or more of the cranial nerves. It is best to give your answer by stating the anatomical abnormality you find (e.g. lower motor neuron lesion of the left VIIth nerve), followed by your evidence for this (as demonstrated by weakness in all facial muscles on the affected side).

The next question is likely to be concerned with the cause(s) of the lesion. It is sensible to start with the commonest (see Chapter 7).

Short case 9: 'Look at this patient – what is the diagnosis?'

This common short case usually means looking at the face. Fear can set in because you are in danger of upsetting the patient as well as the examiner by giving the wrong diagnosis. There are a limited number of conditions in which the face on its own gives the game away:
- thyrotoxicosis
- myxoedema
- acromegaly
- Cushing's disease or syndrome
- Parkinson's disease
- Marfan's syndrome
- Paget's disease

Once you have made the right diagnosis the next question is usually, 'What else would you look for to confirm your diagnosis?' If there is time, the examiner will also ask what investigations you would perform. Make sure you know all the physical signs which you should elicit for each of the above conditions.

The case may not be a 'whole face'. You may only be able to comment on the presence of abnormalities such as xanthelasma, unilateral or bilateral ptosis, unilateral or bilateral exophthalmos or a butterfly rash. Subsequent questions will depend on your correct identification of these features.

Short case 10: 'Look at these hands'

After inspecting the hands for a few moments, ask the patient if they are painful or tender. If the patient is happy for you to proceed, test the power, sensation and fine movements of the hands bearing in mind that you are examining the joints and the nervous system simultaneously. Compare sides as you go.

Common rheumatological diagnoses you might encounter include rheumatoid arthritis (always check the elbows for nodules and the skin for vasculitis), osteoarthritis, psoriatic arthropathy (the typical rash may be visible and the nails may be involved) and gout. Neurological abnormalities which may appear include ulnar, median and radial nerve palsies (see Chapter 7), and peripheral neuropathy. Other conditions which can be diagnosed from examining the hands include systemic sclerosis, carpal tunnel syndrome, acromegaly, Parkinson's disease and Volkmann's ischaemic contracture.

Short case 11: 'Examine the fundi'

This simple case often exposes the candidate's clinical inexperience. Not only are you required to examine the fundus but you also have to work the ophthalmoscope efficiently. A vain attempt at trying to set the ophthalmoscope on the correct lens is an indication to the examiner that you probably don't look into patients' eyes very much.

Start with the ophthalmoscope at + 12 dioptres. Inspect the cornea and lens for cataracts and corneal abrasions. Then 'rack down, until the retina comes into focus. The following conditions are likely:

- hypertensive retinopathy (traditionally grades I to IV: grade I may simply reflect arteriosclerosis and it is therefore better to say 'increased light reflex' rather than 'silver wiring')
- diabetic retinopathy (background and proliferative: diabetic maculopathy and photocoagulation scars may be present)
- optic atrophy
- papilloedema
- glaucoma
- retinitis pigmentosa.

You will usually be asked your findings and then for a diagnosis. There may be clues as to the diagnosis at the bedside: diabetic squash or a bottle of 'BM Stix' for example.

Short case 12: 'Talk to this chap for a few minutes'

This request will confuse a candidate who is not prepared for it and therefore cannot think of an appropriate single question to ask. It is sensible to approach the patient as if he were a long case, first asking his name, age and occupation. Then ask him where he is, the date and time. The patient may be demented but he is more likely to have a dysarthria or dysphasia. Make sure you know the causes of both.

Short case 13: 'Look at this rash'

These cases often appear as 'spot diagnoses' in the exam: the more common skin rashes are the rule. Once you have made your diagnosis you may be asked what other signs you can elicit to confirm it. If, for example, there is psoriasis, you would look at the joints and nails. The rashes encountered will usually be those with 'medical significance' rather than those of purely dermatological interest. You must be able to recognize:

- psoriasis
- eczema
- herpes zoster
- herpes simplex
- systemic lupus erythematosus
- vasculitis
- purpura
- erythema nodosum and marginatum
- neurofibromatosis.

Short case 14: 'Examine this child'

Occasionally children may appear as short cases in the exam. The diagnosis is usually something obvious like Down's syndrome or hydrocephalus, or you may be asked to examine the cardiovascular system. Congenital heart disease would be the commonest abnormality in this respect.

Chapter 6
The Viva

What to expect

During this section, two examiners will question you for a 20 minute period. The topics covered are usually many and varied, and some examiners may have their own X-rays and clinical photographs on which to base their questions. One examiner will first 'occupy the chair' for 10 minutes while the other assesses the candidate's performance. The examiners' roles are then reversed for the second half of the viva.

General preparation

You cannot possibly know what you will be asked so you must practise talking about anything medical. There are two approaches.

Practice oral examinations

Try and persuade a friend, your consultant or almost anyone to quiz you. As the exam approaches you ought to practise answering questions under simulated examination conditions for half an hour per day. Accept the criticisms of your 'examiners' as much as possible and concentrate very hard on making yourself sound interesting, alive and cheerful. Avoid looking terrified and sad. If you are preparing with other candidates, acting as an 'examiner' yourself can give you insight into what impresses or disappoints you about an answer.

Using a pocket dictaphone

You can practise for the exam using this on your own. Jot down a set of likely questions and record your answers: when you play them back you will soon realise whether you are boring, irrelevant or prone to 'errs' and silences. It can also prove very informative if you tape your practice examinations for later review.

There are three important sources of examination questions which you can use during your preparation for the oral:

A textbook

Take a general medical textbook and let it fall open at any page. Whatever heading you see, talk on that subject for two minutes (time yourself properly). If, for example, the page falls open at infective endocarditis discuss it in a logical sequence, stating first of all what the words mean, 'Infective endocarditis is any infection on the inside of a congenital, rheumatic or otherwise damaged heart. The onset is often insidious . . .'. Go through the clinical presentation, pathology, investigations, treatment and prognosis as far as is relevant to the subject. A little practice will help you construct your answers effectively around this simple scheme.

Clinical problems

It is quite common to be given a clinical problem arising from a short case history, and then to be asked to outline how you would approach it. It has been said that the examiners are trying to see how you would manage when your consultant is unavailable. A typical example would be:

'Supposing you are called by the coronary care unit because a patient whom you had admitted earlier in the day with a myocardial infarction had just become extremely dyspnoeic. What would you think of as a possible diagnosis?'

Answer: 'I would go and examine the patient (this is to let the examiner know that you would actually get out of bed), and I would consider an arrhythmia, pulmonary embolus, renal failure, fluid overload (if a drip was running), the onset of pulmonary oedema from left ventricular failure and acute pneumonia.' Having established that you have some idea of the diagnosis the examiners may then ask what investigation(s) you would perform. DO NOT START by suggesting a full blood count but use your commonsense and think what would be useful, i.e. a chest X-ray, and go on from there.

There are a number of texts with examination-type case histories and quite a lot of journals have potted clinical problems which can be used for revision purposes.

The journals

The viva is a favourite time for the examiners to ask about something which has turned up in the journals over the last six months. This particularly refers to the *British Medical Journal*, the *Lancet* and the *New England Journal of Medicine*. Concentrate on leading articles and topical reviews.

During the examination

The comments concerning presentation made in the previous two chapters apply equally to the viva. The examiners will not only be assessing what you say but how it is said. You should aim to be confident and correct as well as succinct. There is no point in trying to circumlocute when asked a question to which you do not know the answer.

Each examiner will have his idiosyncrasies. However, you should remember that the other examiner will be assessing you and may make allowances if he feels that you are not being given the best chance to state your case. Although 20 minutes may seem a short time, the examiners can cover a lot of topics in this period, though you may also be expected to discuss something in depth and at length. Indeed, medical emergencies often serve as a basis for viva questions and you may be required to outline your plan of management in detail.

Typical examination material

Commonly-encountered 'textbook' topics include:

- fibrosing alveolitis
- occupational lung disease
- asthma
- cardiomyopathies
- pericarditis
- cardiac catheterization
- inflammatory bowel disease
- pancreatitis
- gallstones
- Parkinson's disease
- motor neuron disease
- peripheral neuropathy
- systemic sclerosis
- rheumatoid arthritis
- drugs which damage the liver/kidney/lungs

Clinical problems for discussion are similar in many respects to the data interpretation questions in the written part of the exam but here are some examples:

'An elderly lady has an ESR of 110 mm/hr. What would you do?'
'A gentleman complains of substantial weight loss without loss of appetite. What diagnosis do you think of?'
'A patient has an MCV of 102 fl. Why should this be?'
'A female patient aged 20 years has had diarrhoea for three months. What are the possible causes?'
'A patient feels suddenly weak and very unwell in the middle of the night but has no chest pain. The next day there are no abnormal physical findings. What might have happened?'
'An elderly patient is clearly demented. What tests would you perform?'
'A gentleman with a long history of chronic bronchitis is admitted to hospital moribund. Why might he have deteriorated and how would you treat him?'

Some recent topics which have, at the time of writing, appeared in the journals are:
• treatment of the hypothyroid patient with thyroxine – clinical judgement or biochemical control?
• medical complications of pregnancy
• migraine
• lung biopsy
• solvent abuse
• acyclovir
• ketoconazole
• platelets and coronary artery disease
• acquired immunodeficiency syndrome (AIDS)
• coronary angioplasty
• peritoneal dialysis
• exercise and osteoporosis
• benzodiazepines
• heart and lung transplantation
• treating mild hypertension

Chapter 7
Important Examination Lists

Lists are inevitably part of medicine. Those included in this chapter are frequently required, in one form or another, in the answers to questions encountered in all sections of the Part II examination. There is a bias towards neurology because the potential variety of signs makes neurological cases clinical exam favourites.

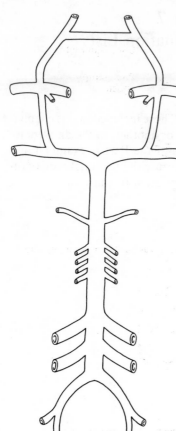

Strokes

Anterior cerebral artery:
- motor and sensory impairment of lower limb more than upper limb
- maybe neural deterioration

Middle cerebral artery:
- hemiplegia (contralateral)
- hemianaesthesia (contralateral)
- aphasia (if dominant hemisphere)
- hemianopia (if optic radiation or internal capsule involved)

Posterior cerebral artery
- Contralateral hemianopia

Vertebro basilar artery
- variable and sometimes transient
- vertigo, facial paraesthesia, dysphasia, drop attacks
- cerebellar signs
- 5th and 10th cranial nerve palsies
- contralateral spinothalamic/pyramidal tract signs

Posterior inferior cerebellar artery
- cerebellar ataxia, nystagmus to side of lesion
- ipsilateral 5th nerve palsy
- bulbar palsy
- contralateral anaesthesia to pain and temperature

Carotid artery
- variable and sometimes transient
- hemiparesis (middle cerebral artery)
- amaurosis fugax

A transient ischaemic attack (TIA) lasts less than 24 hours.

Brown-Séquard syndrome

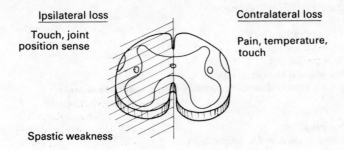

Ipsilateral loss

Touch, joint
position sense

Contralateral loss

Pain, temperature,
touch

Spastic weakness

Syringomyelia

- Pain and temperature loss
- Often motor signs (lower motor neuron type, occasionally upper motor neuron type)

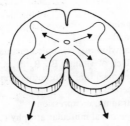

Syringobulbia

Upward extension of the syrinx to involve the lower brain stem leads to dissociated sensory loss on the face, palatal palsy, Horner's syndrome and nystagmus.

Tabes dorsalis

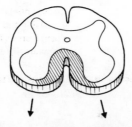

Loss of joint position sense and vibration sense (Dorsal columns)

Pseudobulbar palsy
- Bilateral cranial nerve nuclei affected (upper motor neuron lesion) due to bilateral cerebrovascular events
- Dysarthria
- Difficulty swallowing
- Emotional instability
- Increased jaw jerk
- Mild bilateral hemiplegic signs
- History: Mild unilateral stroke followed by a contralateral stroke

Bulbar palsy
- Unilateral lower motor neuron lesions
- Common causes: Motor neuron disease, encephalitis, vascular lesions
- Dysarthria (12th cranial nerve)
- Difficulty swallowing with regurgitation of fluids through nose.
- Wasting of tongue.
- Death may occur due to pneumonia (inhalation)
- Bulbar symptoms may improve after a rest in myasthenia gravis

Causes of peripheral neuropathy

Metabolic:	diabetes, amyloidosis, chronic uraemia, porphyria
Vitamin deficiency:	lack of vitamin B_1, B_6, B_{12}
Drugs and chemicals:	isoniazid, nitrofurantoin, vincristine, lead, alcohol
Infection:	leprosy
Mechanical:	trauma, compression
Congenital:	peroneal muscular atrophy (Charcot-Marie-Tooth)
Miscellaneous:	polyarteritis, systemic lupus erythematosis, rheumatoid arthritis, carcinoma of the bronchus, Guillain-Barré syndrome

Basal ganglia

Parkinson's disease

Substantia Nigra
- rigidity and akinesia
- tremor at rest, worse if anxious and disappears with rapid movement
- tremor often unilateral
- lack of facial expression
- glabellar tap
- micrographia
- pill rolling of fingers
- festinating gait
- reduced muscle power
- emotional changes

Causes:
- idiopathic – known as paralysis agitans.
- vascular
- post encephalitis
- reserpine
- phenothiazines
- carbon monoxide
- manganese poisoning

Wilson's disease (Hepatolenticular degeneration)

Lentiform Nucleus
- psychiatric changes
- tremor (any type)
- dysarthria
- drooling
- chorea
- akinesia
- rigidity
- dementia
- Kayser-Fleischer Ring
- sunflower cataract

Cause:
disorder of copper metabolism

Chorea

Basal ganglia

Continuous flow of irregular, jerky, explosive movements, flitting from one part to another randomly.

Causes:
- Sydenham's
- Huntington's
- hereditary
- Drug induced
  - neuroleptics
  - phenytoin
  - alcohol
- Hemiballismus (Hemichorea)
  - stroke
  - tumour
  - trauma

Athetosis

Basal ganglia
  (putamen)

Slow, sinuous, writhing movements of the face and limbs most marked peripherally
Grinning face

Causes:
- congenital
- cerebral anoxia at birth

Myopathies

Causes:

Toxic:	Chloroquine, alcohol.
Endocrine:	hyperthyroidism, hypothyroidism, diabetes mellitus, Cushing's syndrome, corticosteroid therapy.
Miscellaneous	hyperkalaemia, hypokalaemia, osteomalacia, carcinomatosis, glycogen storage disease, sarcoidosis.

Myasthenia gravis
(or the carcinomatous myasthenic syndrome)

Signs and Symptoms:
- diplopia, dysarthria, dysphasia,
- difficulty swallowing,
- ptosis.
- Demonstrated by blinking,
  Demonstrated by opening/shutting mouth,
  Demonstrated by clenching/unclenching hand

Test: Intravenous Tensilon (endrophonium hydrochloride)

Muscular dystrophies

Childhood or adolescent
Apparent hypertrophy (fat)

Duchenne type:
- boys, sex-linked recessive,
- latissimus dorsi and pectoralis muscles mainly.
- lordosis,
- waddling gait,
- "climbing up his legs".

Facio-scapulo-humeral type:
- face, shoulder girdle and upper arm.

Limb girdle type:
- Both sexes, autosomal recessive.
- Biceps, triceps, brachioradialis, and lesser extent quadriceps and glutei.

Dystrophia myotonica:
- presents nearer adulthood. Autosomal dominant.
- Facial muscles affected, ptosis common, unable to relax hand.

Wasting of the small muscles of the hand

1 Cord lesions — motor neuron disease
                     syringomyelia
                     tumours
                     cord compression

2 Root lesions — cervical spondylosis
                  neurofibromata

3 Brachial nerve lesions — cervical rib
                           injury

4 Ulnar/Median nerve lesions — injury

5 Disuse atrophy — arthritis

Reflexes:
- ankle jerk L1,2
- knee jerk L3,4
- biceps/supinatus C5,6
- triceps C7,8

Diabetic neuropathy and arteriopathy

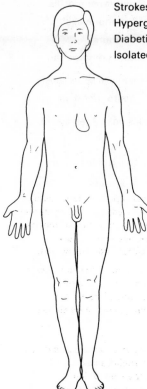

Strokes, dementia
Hyperglycaemic and hypoglycaemic attacks
Diabetic retinopathy
Isolated cranial nerve lesions

Ischaemic heart disease
Ischaemic cardiomyopathy

Autonomic visceral problems

Diabetic amyotrophy
Peripheral atheroma
Painful subacute neuritis
Mononeuritis multiplex
Loss of ankle jerks and vibration sens
Gangrene

Neurological arms

Radial nerve palsy (C5–C8)
- wrist drop, fingers slightly bent
- shaded area of sensory loss

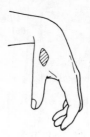

Muscles supplied: triceps, supinatus longus, extensors of wrist, fingers and thumb.

Causes: injury, fractures, pressure from arms over back of chair, injections, crutches, lead poisoning, polyarteritis.

Medial nerve palsy (C6,7,8, T1)
- 'Monkey's hand'. Paralysis grip
- shaded area is sensory loss

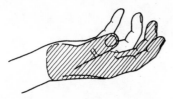

Muscles supplied: long flexors of the forearm, pronatus, two lateral lumbricals, abductor pollicis, opponens pollicis, half flexor pollicis brevis.

Causes: injury, injections, Motor only in poliomyelitis, amyotrophic lateral sclerosis, lead poisoning.

Ulnar nerve palsy (C8, T1)
- 'Claw hand' or 'main en griffe'
- shaded area of sensory loss

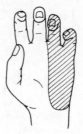

Muscles supplied: flexor carpi ulnaris, medial half of digitorum profundus, hypothenar muscles, medial interossei, medial lumbricals, adductor pollicis.

Causes: injury, fracture, pressure, machine vibrating tools, polyarteritis, leprosy, lead poisoning, leaning on elbows.

Volkmann's ischaemic contracture
- ischaemia causes
  muscle contraction
  throughout the forearm

- Sensory loss in fingers

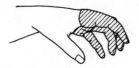

Muscles supplied: long flexors, intrinsic muscles of hand.

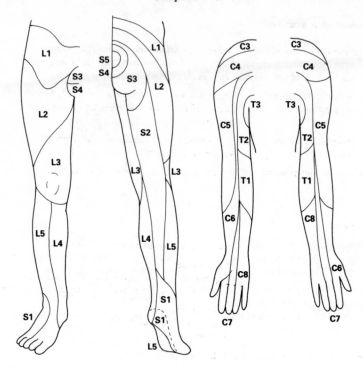

Dermatomes of the legs   **Dermatomes of the arms**

Motor neuron disease

- Progressive muscular atrophy

  Lower motor neuron lesions of the cord are predominant. Fasiculation of muscle. Muscle wasting. Cachexia.

- Amyotrophic lateral sclerosis

  Upper & lower motor neurons affected. Mixed picture of spasticity with progressive muscular atrophy.

- Progressive bulbar palsy

  Motor muscles of medulla & pons. Upper motor neuron signs in arms.

- Pseudo bulbar palsy

  Rarely, upper motor neuron signs predominant.

Tremor

- Rest tremor

  Parkinson's disease.

- Postural

  physiological.
  exaggerated physiological – fear, thyrotoxicosis, alcohol, drugs (antidepressants, lithium, magnesium)

- Intention

  cerebellar, brainstem
  tumours, multiple sclerosis
  vascular lesions.

- Chorea and athetosis are not strictly tremor.

Multiple sclerosis

<50 years – retrobulbar neuritis is commonest presentation
>50 years – progressive wasting of one or more limbs is commonest presentation
also:
- brain stem – transient diplopia
- cerebellar – incoordination of limbs scanning speech
- posterior column loss – electric shock feelings in arm or leg when flexed
- spinothalamic tract lesions – paraesthesia
- bladder – urgency, precipitancy or hesitancy

Neurofibromatosis

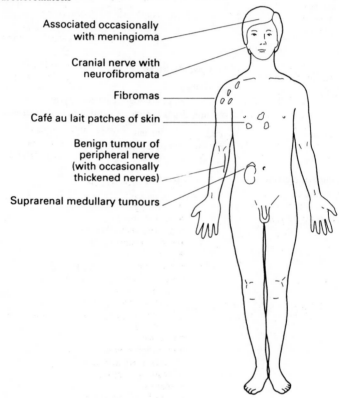

Associated occasionally with meningioma

Cranial nerve with neurofibromata

Fibromas

Café au lait patches of skin

Benign tumour of peripheral nerve (with occasionally thickened nerves)

Suprarenal medullary tumours

Jaundice

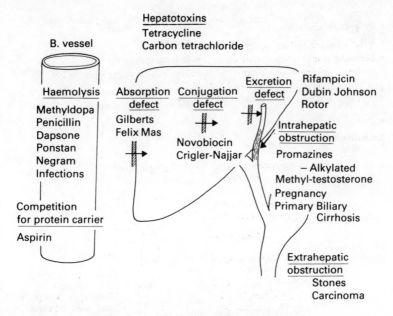

Hepatotoxins
Tetracycline
Carbon tetrachloride

B. vessel

Haemolysis

Methyldopa
Penicillin
Dapsone
Ponstan
Negram
Infections

Competition
for protein carrier

Aspirin

Absorption
defect

Gilberts
Felix Mas

Conjugation
defect

Novobiocin
Crigler-Najjar

Excretion
defect

Rifampicin
Dubin Johnson
Rotor

Intrahepatic
obstruction

Promazines
– Alkylated
Methyl-testosterone
Pregnancy
Primary Biliary
Cirrhosis

Extrahepatic
obstruction
Stones
Carcinoma

Prehepatic coma
● foetor hepaticus
● constructional aprexia
● flapping tremor

Signs of liver failure
● white nails
● clubbing
● liver palms
● proximal myopathy
● scratch marks
● purpura
● bruising
● spider naevi
● yellow sclera
● telangiectasia
● Dupuytren's contracture (alcoholic)
● anaemia
● hair loss
● gynaecomastia
● altered pubic hair
● large liver, spleen
● ascites
● peripheral oedema

Chronic airflow obstruction

Pink puffer
- Progressive dyspnoea of late onset

- Scanty sputum

- Cor pulmonale is usually a terminal event

- $P\text{CO}_2$ normal
- $P\text{O}_2$ normal or slightly reduced

- Thin, energetic, pink dyspnoeic

Blue bloater
- Early onset, repeated attacks

- Profuse sputum

- Cor pulmonale occurs earlier and is commoner

- $P\text{CO}_2$ high
- $P\text{O}_2$ low

- Obese, blue, lazy, not dyspnoeic

Industrial lung disease

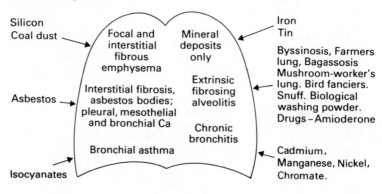

Silicon
Coal dust → Focal and interstitial fibrous emphysema

Mineral deposits only

Iron
Tin

Byssinosis, Farmers lung, Bagassosis Mushroom-worker's lung. Bird fanciers. Snuff. Biological washing powder. Drugs – Amioderone

Asbestos → Interstitial fibrosis, asbestos bodies; pleural, mesothelial and bronchial Ca

Extrinsic fibrosing alveolitis

Chronic bronchitis

Bronchial asthma

Isocyanates →

Cadmium, Manganese, Nickel, Chromate.

Cyanotic congenital heart disease

		Anatomical abnormalities	Physical signs
	Fallot's tetralogy	• ventricular septal defect • right ventricular enlargement • subvalvar pulmonary stenosis • overriding aorta	• cyanosed • systolic murmur over pulmonary outflow tract • right ventricular enlargement
	Tricuspid atresia	• tricuspid valve blocked • ASD or VSD – unless present life is impossible	• cyanosed • systolic murmur across VSD and flow over pulmonary outflow tract • Right ventricular enlargement
	Transposition of the great arteries	• Aorta and pulmonary artery arise from the 'wrong ventricle' • compatible with life only if a shunt is present – usually an ASD or VSD	• cyanosed • systolic murmur of flow or across VSD
	Truncus arteriosus	• a single vessel leads from both ventricles	• cyanosed • systolic flow murmur • Right ventricular enlargement
	Total anomalous venous drainage	• pulmonary veins enter right atrium • compatible with life only if a shunt present. This is usually an ASD or VSD	• cyanosed • systolic murmur across VSD or pulmonary outflow tract • Right ventricular enlargement

LV = Left ventricle RV = Right ventricle LA = Left atrium
RA = Right atrium PA = Pulmonary artery Ao = Aorta
ASD = Atrial septae defect VSD = Ventricular septae defect

Acyanotic congenital heart disease

Atrial septal defect

1° – defect low in septum; often
  involves mitral valve,
2° – defect high in septum

Signs

Wide split fixed second sound

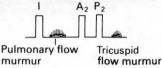

Pulmonary flow   Tricuspid
murmur   flow murmur

Loud pulmonary second sound if
pulmonary arterial hypertension

Ventricular septal defect

large – quiet murmur
small – loud murmur
  – murmur may stop
    before end of systole
    due to muscle closing
    hole: Maladie de Roger

Mitral flow murmur

Murmur across
VSD-pansystolic

Loud pulmonary second sound if
pulmonary hypertension

Patient ductus arterosis

Normally closes after birth due to
prostaglandins. If open may be
helped by indomethacin

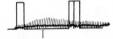

Machinery or   • Collapsing
continuous   pulse
murmur

Coarctation of aorta

Narrowing in aorta is distal
to left subclavian artery

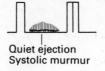

Quiet ejection
Systolic murmur

Hypertension
Delayed and weak
femoral arteries
Murmur between
scapulae
Rib notching on
chest X-ray

Pulmonary stenosis

Valvar or subvalvar
The longer the murmur the
tighter the stenosis

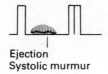

Ejection
Systolic murmur

Enlarged right
ventricle

Selected References

The following books provide useful revision material.

Written paper.

Slide section

Ebden, P., Peiris, M. & Dew, M. (1984) *A Photographic Quiz in Medicine*. Lloyd-Luke, London.

Lester, E. (1982) *MRCP Part 2 Revision Book*. Pastest Service, Hemel Hempstead.

Parfrey, P. & Cramer, B. (1983) *Slide Interpretation in Postgraduate Medicine. Vol. 2. Clinical Signs*. Oxford University Press, Oxford.

Parfrey, P. & Cramer, B. (1983) *X-ray Interpretation for the MRCP*. Churchill Livingstone, Edinburgh.

Parfrey, P. & Cunningham, J. (1981). *Slide Interpretation in Postgraduate Medicine*. Oxford University Press, Oxford.

In addition, the following books produced by Wolfe Medical Publications Ltd (London), are also recommended:

Diagnostic Picture Tests (1984) (Vols. 1–4).

400 Self Assessment Picture Tests in Clinical Medicine (1984).

The Wolfe Medical Atlas series.

Data interpretation

Ashford, R. & Venables, P. (1979) *100 Data Interpretation Questions for the MRCP*. Churchill Livingstone, Edinburgh.

Gabriel, R. & Gabriel, C. (1982) *Medical Data Interpretation for MRCP*. Butterworth, London.

Lester, E. (1982) *MRCP Part 2 Revision Book*. Pastest Service, Hemel Hempstead.

Case histories

Gillmer, M., Gordon, D., Sever, P. & Steer, P. (1979) *100 Cases for Students of Medicine*. Churchill Livingstone, Edinburgh.

Lester, E. (1982) *MRCP Part 2 Revision Book*. Pastest Service, Hemel Hempstead.

Spalton, D., Sever, P. & Ward, P. *100 Case Histories for the MRCP*. Churchill Livingstone, Edinburgh.

In addition, Butterworth (Sevenoaks, Kent) have recently produced a *Case Presentations* series by medical specialty.

Clinicals and orals

Swash, M. & Mason, S. (1984) *Hutchinson's Clinical Methods*. Baillière Tindall, London.

Gupta, K. (1983) *100 Short Cases for the MRCP*. Chapman & Hall, London.
Macleod, J. (1983) *Clinical Examination*. Churchill Livingstone, Edinburgh.

General revision
The following books will prove useful:
British National Formulary (1986) British Medical Association/Pharmaceutical Society of Great Britain.
Burton, J. (1983) *Aids to Postgraduate Medicine*. Churchill Livingstone, Edinburgh.
Gabriel, R. & Gabriel, C. (1983) *Medical Lists for Examinations*. Butterworth, London.
Robinson, R. & Stott, R. (1983) *Medical Emergencies, Diagnosis and Management*. Heinemann, London.
Rubenstein, D. & Wayne, D. (1985) *Lecture Notes on Clinical Medicine*. Blackwell Scientific Publications, Oxford.
Weatherall, D., Ledingham, J. & Warrell, D. (eds) (1983) *Oxford Textbook of Medicine*. Oxford University Press, Oxford.

The following journals are worth regular review:

British Journal of Hospital Medicine
British Medical Journal
Lancet
Medicine Magazine
Nature
New England Journal of Medicine

Index